FROM THE MOUTH
OF THE SUPREME

The Universal and Complete Gift
of Spontaneous Meditation
Specifically for Our Times

By Swami Vishnu Datta

Also by Swami Vishnu Datta
and available from Sanctuary House Press—
WHEN THE SUPREME TAKES A BODY:
The Life of Sri Punitachariji Maharaj

Sanctuary House Press
P. O. Box 332
Crestone, Colorado 81131
www.sanctuaryhouse.org

First Edition
Printed in the United States of America

Cover art: "Datta"
By Marika Popovitz, Crestone, CO

Cover Design: William Howell

Library of Congress Cataloguing-in-Publication Data
Datta, Swami Vishne

From the Mouth of the Supreme:
The Universal and Complete Gift of
Spontaneous Meditation Specifically for Our Times

ISBN 0-9761737-0-0   (pbk: alk. paper).

1. Meditation   2. Lord Dattatreya
3. Spiritual Journey   4. Consciousness

For all who seek the Fullness
that merges Truth and Love in the complete human being.

May the constant rain of blessings
from the heart of Life, Light and Love
be consciously integrated and expressed through each of us.

CONTENTS

PART III   A HANDFUL OF CLARITIES

PART IV *SADANA*: PRACTICE and PRACTICALITIES

PART V   QUESTIONS

PART VI   EXPERIENCES

PART VII   *HARI OM TATSAT JAI GURU DATTA* IN THE WEST

APPENDIX

Author's Forward

We live, despite mountains of evidence to the contrary, in an intensely spiritual age. Life in its fullness is clearly interested in supporting its own essence and expression wherever and however the drive for fullness is present. This book is a testament to precisely this assertion.

The Divine gift presented in these pages was given for our very times. Into daily alarms in the media, into the angst created by political and cultural alienation, into the fear of retreating into a protected past or leaping adventurously toward an unknown future, into the threat of human annihilation at the very time in which a true human family is possible has come something very potent and very practical to guide us into the layered dreams of the heart that announce the cause of love. The Supreme is doing everything possible to assist us in this critical phase transition from one state of human development to a more harmonious and interconnected state. Given that humanity is hungry for true nourishment that will feed both our knowledge and our direct experience, the most powerfully blessed spiritual tool possible in these times has been bestowed. It comes directly from the Source of Revelation and has been designed for everyone, without regard to color, caste or creed.

Since the opening of the 20th century, when time was seen to be relative and no longer a given, our world has found itself in the greatest global shift in recorded human affairs. The demands of this period already are profoundly challenging and profoundly promising, a motion that will only accelerate, producing an astonishing degree of change. A 1990's *Time Magazine* poll of the ten deepest fears ranked

'change' at the top of the list. How we live with change is a
question that is already assuming a daily relevance.

Key to our era is our understanding of
interconnectedness. Human ecology is no different than the
web of life woven so intricately in the natural world, which
teaches that every species is an important part of the whole.
We are all related. Indeed, we are at least as unified as we are
different. No matter where we live, whatever the climate or
culture, regardless of our status or beliefs, we each want to
love and be loved, we want to belong and to be happy. Yet
the question comes: Is what we want really possible?

This query arises from the universal need in each of us
to be connected to our own self, so that our strength— rather
than trying to hold onto the myriad shifting requirements of
work, society and family—is first and foremost secured by an
inner confidence that moves compassionately and consistently
through all the demands of our lives.

Beckoning us through the door opening onto new
possibilities for individual and collective human development
is this universal gift offered precisely for our changing,
challenging, promising era. It takes simplicity to a new
dimension and profundity to its limit, at the same time
bringing tremendous protection and maturing integration.
For anyone longing for the fullness of self, reality, expression
and capability, this gift brings unprecedented blessings and
makes the life we each hold most truly in our hearts not only
possible but also deeply rich.

Just one of the many blessings of this Divine gift
is the state of meditation—sought after by so many yet
not necessarily granted even after years or decades of
practice. Given the dozens or even hundreds of meditation

methodologies and practices, why is the meditation described in this book important? Because, regardless of method, there still remains the question: How do I meditate? That query is answered by Spontaneous Meditation—which, beyond any method or technique, allows the state of meditation to happen naturally, automatically and spontaneously. This stunningly simple and yet most complete and safe spiritual gift requires no shift in belief or dress or allegiance. Just using this tool will bring whatever your life requires, including the passion and peace, the wisdom and humor to gracefully negotiate the shifting and uncharted terrains of our quickening modern era.

Feeling a lasting responsibility to our human family and knowing the potential of these times, I offer what was given to me by the one through which this gift originated. In that gift—which understandably appears too good to be true—I stand in its certainty: What you really want *is* possible, and herein you will receive the simplest and most blessed way of moving toward that happiness.

Your life is the unique expression of Life itself. If you are authentic in reaching the full beauty of who you are, I invite you inward.

Vishnu Datta
Crestone, Colorado
August 2004

PART I

THE GIFT

*All I want is for those who are searching
for the Truth to find something real.*

— Bapu —

Introduction

You may well have entertained the mythic question which has piqued human consciousness for ages unknown: "If I had one wish—what would it be?"

If you are asking for material possessions, you might place yourself before a proverbial genie. If you are requesting spiritual gifts, you might imagine yourself before a great sage. If, however, your wish is for all humankind, then only the Author of Creation could grant such a boon.

While asking the Divine for a wish may seem the stuff of legend, it did happen to someone in 1975. This possibility was given to a great personage, whose affectionate name is 'Bapu', a true yogi saint as yet largely unknown in the West.

To ask something of the Supreme, one boundary must be observed: the free will of others cannot be altered. Therefore, what may seem to be the noblest of wishes—the ending of poverty, hunger and disease in our human family— is not permissible. Given this understanding, we see that what the Divine could bestow would be an idea for a system of knowledge or service, an invention or tool that could potentially change the world. Such was given to Bapu.

Rather than wishing for anything for himself, this wisest of persons wished for something for all of humanity, for all of us. Bapu asked for the most potent and user-friendly tool possible for human fulfillment, especially for our times when individuals are starving for a way they can be nourished throughout all their bodies—spiritual, emotional, mental and physical.

Let us inquire objectively at the outset of this book,

what would constitute the optimum spiritual tool? What qualities would a tool have that was gifted to humanity by the Divine?

The optimum spiritual tool would be for everyone, regardless of class or culture, creed or constitution.

We would want it to be simple to use, without guesswork, without dependence on our IQ or social connections or economic capability.

And would we not want this gift to be free, without cost, without any strings attached?

We would want this tool to be complete, that using it would not require other tools later on, that this tool would be the only one needed for our growth.

Moreover, we would want such a tool to work... every time we use it.

We would expect the optimum spiritual tool to be safe, fully protective and integrating, so that one part of ourselves would not develop faster or slower than other parts, thereby avoiding the pitfalls of unbalanced growth.

We would hope it would be potent, powerful, capable of bringing grace and ease, strength and awareness to any and all issues we would

want to address. In a word, we would want it to
lead to our happiness.
And who wouldn't it to be a continuous gift, that
we would receive continually for as long as life
lasts and assist us as far as we could want to
go, in this life and beyond?

We would want to be able to become more
ourselves, not like someone else, but to become
more unique and also more universal.

And, returning to our first criterion, we would
hope that this gift not require us to change our
dress or address, our job or interests, and not
tamper with our beliefs.

If a spiritual tool could be that universal and available, that strong and also that gentle—attentive to the uniqueness of each of our lives so that we could travel with it in all the ways that we require—then we may well be able to call it an ultimate spiritual tool. Such a tool is the basis of this handbook.

However, given this stunning possibility, we should not expect the journey of life to become an effortless jaunt to fullness. While this boon, a miracle given to us all, comes as close to a guarantee as is possible in spiritual development—it is not miraculous. It does require our participation, our sincere spiritual practice. The only way to know this gift is to try it, to experience and test it.

1. Having Taken a Precious Human Body...

Here we are!
The breezes swirl around and rustle our branches, yet inside
Our limbs and trunk churns the hurricane of longing light.
We are that rush, that breath, that ever-yearning silent sap.

—Vishnu Datta—

The amazing process of being birthed into this realm of space, time, gravity, meaning, mobility and the five senses has us on a great adventure whose goal is not specified on our birth certificate. Our parents may or may not have pointed to the finish line, if indeed there is one. And there are no maps for sale in the super markets. We see that some souls appear to be gifted with insight, others with vision or perseverance, while many others seem uninspired.

Regardless of our upbringing, social standing and education or lack of it, we know that life is not all that we want. We know we suffer and have contributed to the suffering of others. We likely sense that this life on Earth is something of a school and that there is a purpose why we are enrolled.

Our educational system has, at the time of this writing, still not adjudicated 'Happiness' as part of the course of study, let alone the core thrust of its curriculum.

While some of us find encouragement from the voices of society and many others reap only discouragement, even if we do rise to what our friends may unanimously term 'success,' we are not guaranteed an inner feeling of completeness. We may have any number of Ph.Ds and still be miserable. "We are only two swings out of the jungle," says one of my mentors with a smile.

All this difficult insight is rising because of the inherent longing of the human spirit to unfold its essence. This is an intensely spiritual age. And, if in the face of such repressiveness we still sincerely are interested in the possibility of happiness, then we want to live, not just to survive, and we want to belong in a satisfying way to our human family. But happiness is not a commodity that we, at some point, get enough of. Rather, we all want to be happier, which is to say that we will not be satisfied until we have, in a sense, become as full as life itself, until we no longer carry on our shoulders or in our hearts the burden of separation.

This 'unitive dimension' beyond separation—of becoming all that this school can teach us—is the primal urge of every soul. In some persons this drive gets interpreted in such limited ways, from addictions to criminality, as to bring pain to self and others, whereas this drive moves other souls to historic levels of service and even to the infinite realm of Love.

The Divine gift of this book speaks directly to why we each uniquely have taken a body and to the fulfillment of those natural longings that come with our breath and heartbeat.

2. The Challenge and Possibility of Our Amazing Era

We could not have chosen more beautifully
Than to now appear from the damp soil of our mother.
We are designed to wake up in this stalk of love.
To wake and revision what it means to grow and flower.

—Vishnu Datta—

We are alive in what will likely prove the most astounding period in recorded history, in which human existence itself is threatened, while simultaneously a true family of humanity arises not just as a definite possibility, but as a necessity. These, indeed, are watershed times. The entire course of human enterprise, of civilization itself, has on every level been gushing out of immaturity and fear for millennia. Now that great river, significantly shifting its direction during the last century, will flow out of motivations far more caring and creative than before, which is to say that the values—the bedrock underneath every thought and action—of human behavior are shifting. The tectonic plates of the collective psyche are in motion, because of the willingness of a great number of souls—though they as yet constitute a somewhat small percentage of our human race— to shift their inner beliefs and attitudes. This shift in energy will produce a far-ranging shift in action and in the forms of human exchange.

The identification of our lives with issues of security, pleasure/esteem, and power/control has placed our race on a trajectory of disaster. The urge to protect ourselves, the tendency to avoid pain, the deflection away from integrity due to insincere and even violent attitudes, and the need to be tough and affluent on behalf of 'number one' at the expense of others have disabled our inherent capacities for innocence, trust and vulnerability. Humanity is in a time of crisis, so elegantly defined by its Chinese ideogram as 'Danger' over 'Opportunity'.

The script for the theater of life on Earth is, nevertheless, wondrously written. Our global predicament is designed to move souls to look into the reason for being in a body. This is a clarifying age, a gateway, a door into stunning arenas of harmony. A phase transition—as when water boils to move from a liquid to a gas—is already well under way. Humanity is likewise changing states, from one bound to limitation toward one aimed at vast possibility—from ignorance toward knowledge, from exclusivity toward inclusivity, from violence toward peace; from separateness toward interconnectedness; from fear toward love. Ours is a most fortunate time to be alive.

Yet ours is a most challenging time, as well. Change—that most feared human arena, mysterious yet universal—is upon us to a degree that is designed to exceed every expectation. Society may well be like the sultan who, interviewing a number of artisans to create a mosaic floor in a proposed addition to his palace, naively hires the cheapest, an artist who charges a penny the first day, doubling every day for a month. Because it has cost him only 64 cents by week one and barely $40 by week two, the sultan doesn't see that on day 30 he will have paid nearly $10,000,000. If our world changed in this way—beginning, say, in 1990 with a mere 1% shift—we would be experiencing a strong but negotiable 164% difference as this book is being written, but a nearly 5,000,000% shift by 2020.

To deal with unprecedented change will require a sense of centeredness, a stability that originates not primarily within some nation or corporation or even family—but within ourselves. The paradigm shift of our age is meant to reveal our human beingness, why we are here and who we are as individuals. Yet, our worldwide state of affairs requires not only self-awareness, but also global awareness. Are we prepared to accept as our sister and brother every other soul, no matter his or her color or creed or homeland or status? We are in the process of finding out that on this spinning planet we are all connected, are all interdependent, are all related.

Freedom and harmony, the issues of our age, are not antithetical. How free we want to be is also to ask, "How free do we want to be from harming others?" How much freedom and harmony is possible? We each have to ask and answer that question ourselves. We know that separation constitutes the foundation of fear, so that the degree of freedom and harmony we long for is equivalent to how much separation we are willing to overcome by seeing it as mere illusion.

Coming to the integrity of uniting freedom and harmony is not a motion separate from our living. Life itself is set up for exactly what we want. It is time to shift our attention, our values and dedications toward that which we each desire. For this we have been born. For this the world is mysteriously changing and shifting toward a unitive dimension that holds and nurtures all diversity while preserving commonality. We are each a universe. We each are individual and immense. We each require guidance, because we each require fullness. In actuality, we are the fullness that we long for—but we need to find out for ourselves, in actual and direct experience coupled with certain knowledge, that such, indeed, is the case. In this time and specifically for this time, a simple spiritual tool to accomplish all the freedom and harmony we desire has been given to anyone who is so moved.

3. Our Mysterious Journey to Certainty

No one has gone far.
The road turns again and again out of sight.
We learn to move by moving on When each step is my first,
I have become my walking.

—*Vishnu Datta*—

We are in the greatest of all stories. This one-of-a-kind sojourn to the very purpose of life is a trek to our very own self. Navigation requires both knowledge and experience. To become conscious that we are travelers is to deeply recognize that our life has meaning.

The good news and bad news of our journey can be summed up in a single sentence: We have infinite dreams and apparently only finite resources to satisfy those dreams.

We are blessed with free will—to choose our path, our dream, our destination. Yet we may feel overwhelmed by the hugeness of so many possibilities. Some of us may leap over all sorts of obstacles to enact a vision that mirrors life's vastness, while others of us may feel intimidated into focusing on some very doable routine, something that minimizes mystery and risk. No matter our response to the ten thousand demands that naturally arise as a result of having being born, that which brought us to life is interested in our being alive. We could say that life itself has a built-in bias in favor of our expressing the potential stored within us. It is as if the life of Creation 'out there' and our inner life bubbling up 'in here' want to communicate, want to fall in love. It is love that reveals the 'out there' and the 'in here' to be one and the same.

Yet life unfolds, level by level, as meaning expands and deepens with each layer we traverse. How layered is our human existence? The numerous sedimentations of the Grand Canyon give a hint. Each stratum, like each person, has its peculiar gifts and purposes, and each, like each person, requires a new understanding and a corresponding energy adjustment.

'Life', 'God', 'Reality', 'Love', 'the Universe'— however we name that intelligence of truth and vitality responsible for our existence—is infinitely adept in orchestrating the symphony by which each of us in our own way and pace comes to fullness. To factor in the actuality of our utter uniqueness is to glimpse how unfathomable is the great dance we all are in, how vast the dance floor, how varied the music, how many the ways to move in our response to being human.

The journey to fullness we each will experience has never been experienced exactly as we will live it! Some of us will walk, some will ride a bicycle, some will drive a car, some will take a train, and some will fly by jet. We cannot have every possible experience. But the vistas we each will witness reveal exactly the terrain we require for our specific destiny.

Our travels begin to mysteriously uncover a sense that life exists as a series of veils, and that neither the mind nor the heart, by themselves, will penetrate with integrity the illusion that each veil portrays. To pass through a veil requires that we receive the message encoded in its reality. Moving one by one beyond the limited energetic of any veil or boundary is part of our individual pilgrimage toward the certainty of love.

How far into that certainty will we each travel? It is said that some have heard of the sea, some have seen it, some have smelled it, some have tasted it, some have waded in it, some have swum in it, and some have even drowned in it and so have *become* the sea. The question arises: "How intimate with the ocean of existence do I want to be?"

To the degree that we move through these veils, we come into deeper relationship with paradox, which exists in order that we see beyond reason, beyond cause and effect, beyond the intellect, beyond limitation and pairs of opposites. Life is an art—the deepest of all arts. All art begins with seeing—with the insight that comes from our internal sense of self meeting with our unique sense of self-expression. That which we truly see we truly become. If we become what we see, what then will transform limited seeing into the truest of insight and vast capacity for vista? What will open my eyes the widest?

We all want to know what this journey of journeys will look like. The image of climbing the sacred mountain may be helpful. First, we hear of this mountain. Maybe we even see it. At some point we may be moved to climb it. We will be wise to first study about the climb—to read about unexpected weathers, study the many types of knots and research the best tent and backpack available. Here, book knowledge can be valuable. Once we are prepared, the climb itself begins—which is totally experiential. Despite the maps we might bring, our ascent will be unique: No one has climbed or will climb the sacred mountain quite like we will. If we can navigate shifting terrains and environments and make it above tree line, we will with diligence and faith reach the peak. There, beyond all paths and rules and rituals, we will stand in true religion, which is none other than our union with the Divine. But this is not the final 'summit'. One more great step beckons us: that we come down the mountain and re-enter society, where our task is, with every step and breath, to find in the marketplace all that we were graced to enjoy at the pinnacle of the sacred mountain.

Our journey will resemble every other journey, for we are universal beings, which is to say that all our journeys are fundamentally the same—out of bondage and into freedom. Yet concomitantly we are one-of-a-kind beings, meaning that, though wise to navigate with the map that reveals the nature of the journey itself, we will have to trust enough to authentically enact whatever path we choose so that it becomes *our* path, *our* life as life has never before been expressed. And, since we never solve the mystery of life (except by becoming the mystery), we learn how to journey only by making the journey.

Because such a saga can seem overwhelming or even impossible, the Divine gift to encourage every possibility to completeness is presented in Part II.

4. The Delicate and Powerful Issue of Religion

Oh my God! How amazing
That nothing said about You is true.
Only finding You myself will make sure
You are beyond all words, Your secret ever safe with me.

—*Vishnu Datta*—

Religion represents the deepest impulse in the human breast—to answer all of life's questions by *becoming* all that life is—which constitutes the realm of human fulfillment. If any soul were to be utterly complete by any means whatsoever, then that means would qualify as 'religion,' which literally means 'to bind back.' To make a conscious return to our natural self beyond temporal and spatial boundaries, to utterly belong, to come to fullness, to finally be non-separate, to unite with the origin of Being and Creation—this is the most primal and subtlest urge in our being. More subtle than religion is Religion, the centrality of Reality. Understanding the principle—that what is most subtle is most powerful—is important. To simply break open a clock with a hammer destroys the possibility of telling time. However, to break open a clock at its subtlest level—beyond even its atomic existence—would create enough energy to light the world. Prior to every religion is Religion, the trunk of all the paths of return to the Source. To access the realm of Religion within us is to dwell in the most nutritious, healthy and original strata of ourselves, and from there our cups naturally overflow.

Religion expresses the unitive dimension of life in which all the diversities and differences of individual expression are aligned in knowledge, peace, love and mercy. It is the ken of religion to help us organically respond to the big questions (for example, "Who am I?") which especially arise in an age such as ours. It is the agency of religion which is designed to address our crises, especially the crisis of identity.

Yet how strange that the very field whose fertility offers lasting freshness, beauty, interconnectedness and knowledge has historically become the terrain on which so much warfare and lack of love has been displayed. Such is the power of human consciousness—to unite and to separate, to reveal and to limit.

Into the already incandescent issues of religion—hot because they are powerful and represent our longing to most deeply belong—enters the notion of God. No name can accurately portray or contain that which 'God' is meant to stand for. Thus it is that God is all too often regarded and reduced to a concept, one that has seemed to both uplift and complicate human existence. For this reason, Lord Buddha did not even refer to God, but avoided the many over-arching questions whose answers come only once we know our own nature: Is there a God and, if so, is there one or are there many? Is God real or created? Is God wrathful or benign? Is God available, interested in human affairs, interested in 'me'? Is God attainable or will there always be separation? Was anything before God? Is God in a form or beyond form? Such inquiries have both inspired and plagued the enactment of human history.

Whatever has engendered and holds together Creation must be common to all that exists in this universe and in all universes, if there are more than one, and, therefore, essential and simple enough to be ultimate and unitive. God must be that which is true and real in all times and places and dimensions. By definition, that which is worthy of the loftiest word in any language must be all-powerful, all-knowing and everywhere present, utterly without partners, yet whose 'government' perfectly orchestrates all Creation down to the fall of a sparrow, as Shakespeare's Hamlet learned. God, infinitely beyond form, has taken every form, yet must be indivisible. Having created, God is also the relationship which we call 'love', for God holds together every particle and thought and action of every being in Creation.

The Oneness of all diversity, loving every creation, does not judge—we invented that trick ourselves—and has no preference for which path we choose, or which name we give to the Ultimate—only that we travel with integrity to where we most want to go. Thus, the 'problem' with God lies completely with us.

Standing on the shore and enamored with the floating multiplicities of Creation, we do not directly experience the Ocean of Life, even though the vastness of this water is our very own nature. Though such purity, depth and endless expansiveness are inseparable from our natural state, thousands of years of 'civilization' have engrained in us countless attachments to a world that seems 'out there' and, therefore, separate. The issue, therefore, is not God as God is, but ourselves who have so poorly interpreted God into an array of concepts that God is not.

All of the great spiritual traditions of our planet arose out of Divine unity, and each was designed to return us to our original state of oneness with Life itself. Each of our great spiritual traditions was born in a definite geography, climate and socio-political context. Thus, they are all like wells—in the forest, at the foot of a mountain, near a stream, in the desert—into the same underground bounty of water. They each are diamonds favoring their own most cherished facet of the Divine: Knowledge is the Hindu/Vedic preference, obedience for Jews, peace for Buddhists, love for Christians, and surrender for Muslims. Because all the religions of our planet were born in the originality of Divine power, truth, compassion, beauty and humility—the wisdom of revealed traditions which have guided souls for centuries can be a great friend and a consistent blessing. All these traditions are great, yet over time have come into limited interpretations long since interwoven with their respective cultures, such that even well-meaning souls, given the historical conflicts seemingly inherent in religion, often reject what is supposed to be a divine inheritance. Says Bapu, "Religions have built walls and it is time these walls come down."

It is only recently that our human family has all religions at its fingertips. In our global community, we see that our religious traditions are inter-related. And we sense, until they each can sit with one another in a circle of harmony, that the peace we long for as a human family will be impossible. We will not feel at ease within ourselves until the most subtle and powerful impulse within us comes to rest, until the great religions not only tolerate one another, but also act with respect and even admiration towards their sisters and brothers of other persuasions. And, while there exists a hope in many hearts that all these religions should simply come together in mutual unity, our age is one not just of differences or just of unity, but of unity in diversity. This is the meaning of 'uni-verse'. The co-existence of religious unity and diversity demands more consciousness and more maturity than mere unity. Such is the call of our unprecedented times.

5. The Most Inter-religious Place on Earth

I want to live
Where the eye has no judgment
And the ear delights in dancing to every hymn.
There, taking the lap of any lover as my home,
   I will be at home everywhere.

—*Vishnu Datta*—

To not be inter-religious, at least in a mutuality of respect, is to not be a human family. This is why the Lord of Lords, in presenting to Bapu the Divine gift of our times, chose the most inter-religious place on Earth.

Thoughts may go to Jerusalem or other multi-religious cities, but the place where this gift was bestowed was at the foot of one of India's three most sacred mountains: Mount Girnar. What is important about Mount Girnar is not that it rises out of the west-central India plain in the state of Gujarat to a height of some 4,000 feet; or that it is a most unusual mountain, having nine peaks rising out of formidable rock; or that its edifice clearly reveals the face of a sage; or that it is a sacred pilgrimage site with 5,000 steps leading to the top and 5,000 more leading to Lord Datta's footprints in stone, the path up the mountain being lined with temples, both Hindu and Jain, some more than 1000 years old.

What is important is that this fortress-like mountain is hollow inside—we cannot see this fact with ordinary eyes. Caves and conference rooms abound within its hidden spaces, for Girnar is home to the *Siddhas* (perfected beings) who guide and guard all the religions and sacred paths that lead to fullness of life. In the inner caves and conference centers—seen only with the inner eye—the *Siddhas* do their *sadhana* (spiritual practice, the root of this word meaning 'to accomplish') and gather to discuss *yoga* (the way to lasting union with God and Reality) and the future of humanity.

Mount Girnar symbolizes a place where the Source of humanity and all the currents and religions of human longing converge. It is no accident that Bapu met the Supreme at the foot of Mt. Girnar, and that this mantra is offered to all humanity—as a practice in itself or as a powerful addition to any practice in which a seeker of any persuasion already has faith. All the religions, all the spiritual paths and beliefs are contained and honored in this mantra.

6. The Oneness of the Three Faces

See, the clouds have one sky mother.
Listen: Every note of music begins and ends in silence.
Hah! I have been lied to since my birth...
Each flower in the garden is the greatest.

—Vishnu Datta—

The Divine gift was presented at the foot of Mount
Girnar, a mountain mentioned in the ancient Vedic texts as
Rejavak and sacred to Lord Dattatreya. *Treya* means 'three',
referring to the three faces of Lord Dattatreya, for Lord Datta
is the fusion of the three primal energies of Creation: the
Generative force, the Operative force and the Destructive
force: G-O-D. *Datta* (the short form of 'Dattatreya') means
'the One Who gives everything away'. This is great news:
The Lord of Lords wants to give everything to us!

Lord Datta is Sadguru, the Essence of all wisdom
traditions throughout time, the utter source and distillation
of all that has been taught by every messiah, avatar, seer,
prophet, sage or saint. If all the religious traditions of the
world were spokes in a wheel, Lord Dattatreya would reside
in the very center of the hub, the source and common meeting
point of all the spokes. Though humans often tend to feel
their chosen religion to be the best, the wheel of Life depends
on all the spokes.

Lord Datta is understood to have three faces, though,
actually, the Supreme is beyond all form. This form simply
depicts the power that God, by definition, must hold. Any
divine form is but a symbolic portrayal of all that lives
beyond depiction, beyond description and concept. Lord

Datta is beyond all form, yet has appeared to those fortunate enough to have his/her *darshan* (presence).

Understanding the spiritual contribution that has come from Lord Datta specifically for our times resides in our appreciation of its source—the unity of Lord Brahma (the Creator), Lord Vishnu (the Maintainer) and Lord Shiva (the Destroyer), according to the Vedic tradition. This creation, this maintenance and this destruction are constantly occurring on every dimension from vast to minute—from the smallest of the small to the largest of the large. Physicists have for some time identified the three mathematical operators present in every action: the creative, the maintaining, and the destructive. In other words, Generation, Operation and Destruction are present in every moment and action in Creation. The One Who is the completeness of Generation, Operation and Destruction throughout this and every universe is G-O-D, is God. Lord Datta holds together throughout every dimension and time the three mathematical operators of every action.

Is God one or a committee? If a committee, then the head of the committee deserves the name *God*. Bapu has said that all the gods and goddesses (all the laws of nature, for each divine personage represents a clear structure and function of Creation) chose Lord Dattatreya to have "the onerous distinction" of being "the Guru of Gurus", that is to say being the head of all the divine intelligences and all the fulfilled human beings whose job it is to share all that they have been given. Every deity, every law of nature, issues forth from the Three-in-One, the Vedic Trinity. In Christian terms, Lord Brahma represents the Son, Lord Vishnu the Holy Spirit, and Lord Shiva the Father. Every aspect and intelligence of Creation and the Source of Creation must gain Lord Dattatreya's permission to carry out any action. And, since representations of the Godhead are just that—representations—we can understand Lord Dattatreya as being equivalent to the Divine Mother, Who is the Unitive and Trinitarian fullness of life as seen through the feminine lens.

Lord Datta is the very highest and most all-encompassing source—omnipresent, omnipotent, and omniscient and incorporating all pairs of opposites. All spiritual paths meet in Sadguru Datta, Who is classically portrayed as having not just three faces, but also six arms, each bearing a symbol of Divine potency. Usually, these are understood to be a discus, which can slay all negativity; a trident, symbol of Lord Shiva; a flower, symbol of all that is beautiful and rooted and is growing toward the light; a conch, which blows the original note of Creation (OM, the first sound, holding in its nature the beginning, middle and end of all that exists); a mace, indicating authority and that power which can overcome any obstacle; and a *mala* (rosary) which stands for *sadhana* (spiritual practice) and all the ways of remembering the Lord so that we return union with the Divine.

Lord Dattatreya is traditionally pictured sitting on a rock, which is covered with a deerskin (symbol of Liberation), left foot on the ground and the right leg crossed to the left knee—indicating that the Lord of Lords is both standing on the earth as well as seated in meditation posture. Important companions of the Lord are a white cow and four dogs. The cow is well-accepted to be a sacred animal in India and stands for forgiveness and compassion. The cow gives everything—milk, curds and its dung, which is used for everything from fuel to building houses and from carrying out ceremonies to making medicines—and keeps on giving. The dogs stand for the important qualities of attentiveness, loyalty, obedience and companionship. In India, they are among the lowest of creatures, part of the garbage disposal system. Therefore, the dogs convey the magnanimity of the Lord, signifying that the Divine is fully for every creature, even the lowliest. Moreover, the dogs represent the four Vedas, the four main books of Vedic literature that deal with the knowledge of the absolute nature of Reality (*Rig Veda*) , the art of living in the interface of the Absolute with the relativity of rhythm and form (*Sama Veda*), the vast fields of health—from being free from sickness to being free from negativity—and how to live without suffering (*Yejur Veda*), and the relative arenas of science, mathematics, wealth and the like (*Artharva Veda*). *Veda* means 'knowledge,' full knowledge. Thus, if the subject were a flower, the Veda would speak of the flower and leaves and stem, and also of the root; and not only of itself, but also of its companion plants and animals and insects; and not only of the various weathers and soils, but also of the wind, sun, moon and stars and their influences—ergo, the completeness of the knowledge of the source, course and goal of life in a flower. The Vedas are the oldest records of human experience, written in ancient Sanskrit, a divinely given language. It is called *Devanauguri*, which means 'Divine tongue,' and, according to many scholars, constitutes the root of all the languages of our planet. The gift coming from the Lord would, therefore, be *Veda* and would contain all favors and all knowledge.

Dattatreya did actually incarnate into human form. In his incarnation as the sixth *avatar* (Divine incarnation) of Lord Vishnu, Datta had 24 gurus—the sun, moon, mountain, bird, bee, prostitute, etc.—for He learned from every experience; all of life revealed its importance to Him. And, while often appearing as a madman, He never forgets anyone who prays to Him. The name 'Datta,' means "The one who gives away everything"—all his possessions (knowledge) and even his very own Self. Indeed, throughout the ages, to those most surrendered devotees Lord Dattatreya has even bestowed His own form, not that such adepts have three faces and six arms, but that they are in such mystic union with the Lord that they feel they do. To Bapu, who has surrendered completely, the Lord has given everything. Through the Divine gift bestowed on November 15, 1975, Sadguru Datta as given to Bapu the most powerful and effective spiritual tool for human happiness. What Bapu received constituted the best avenue in which the Lord could give Himself away.

Despite all that can be written about Lord Dattatreya, Bapu quotes an ancient sage, "No one can say anything about Datta," meaning the Supreme is beyond all description, all elucidation, all understanding.

7. Forty Years

To run and run and go on running—
If I come to love running—
Means having given up the goal for the going.
I am certain then of arriving at the purpose of all roads.

—Vishnu Datta—

The Divine does not simply wave a wand, thereby
healing the human race, but rather works through our
humanity, through great souls who long for the fulfillment of
other souls. Life uses the human to reveal the Divine. On
the slopes of Mount Girnar, a virtually secret yogi saint lived
alone for 12 years. He performed *sadhana* 18 hours a day
in a cave three feet tall and wide and six feet long. His only
companions were monkeys and lions, though occasionally
someone passed by and left a bit of food. That alone he
would eat, due to a vow he had made many years earlier
toward the beginning of his own journey.

It was on the banks of the Narmada River, one of
India's most sacred rivers. This aspirant, who now bears
the name of Shri Punitachariji Maharaj and is affectionately
called 'Bapu' had longed to see a vision of Lord Krishna. He
had been magnetized to the Himalayas, but on route there was
internally guided to Gujarat in west-central India. He had
left a deeply successful life as a *pujari* (one who conducts
the many categories of ritualistic Vedic ceremonies), and a
reciter of the Indian epics, such as the *Ramayana* (the story
of Lord Ram and his wife Sita, who is stolen by Ravanna,
a ten-headed demon). Having come to the Malsar, Bapu
took up residency in an uninhabited temple sacred to Lord

Shiva. He decided he would serve the Lord in this place and be content to be served by the Lord. Thus it was that Bapu took a vow to eat only that food the Lord would provide, which meant he would eat only whatever might be offered to the Lord in this temple. That very evening a man brought several stramonium fruit and placed them at the feet of the Lord. Such fruits, while constituting an acceptable gift to Lord Shiva, are poisonous to humans. Given the vow he had made, Bapu—though he knew the nature and effects of such a fruit—put his entire life into the Lord's hands and went ahead and ate. As predictable, he began to die. Later that night a wandering saint came by who knew what had happened, and this man administered an antidote, thereby saving Bapus' life. Yet Bapu continued his vow.

From the banks of the Narmada, said to give its blessings to those who even look at its waters (whereas one has to bathe in the Ganges and cross the Yamuna to gain the favors of those two sacred rivers), Bapu was inwardly directed to Mount Girnar. There he lived in three caves, the first two no longer existing (the latter one destroyed by water). The third cave, where he spent the final years of his dedication to the Lord, is still intact and just a 45-minute hike from Girnar Sadhana Ashram, where Bapu resides at the foot of Mount Girnar.

It was 1973 when Bapu was guided down the mountain, at the urging of several aspirants who had discovered this great yogi saint and wanted to build him an ashram. Bapu, as a result of his years on Mount Girnar, had become an acknowledged *dende swami*, the highest form of renunciate.

In a film of the current ashram, far more spacious and

welcoming than the original thatched hut and small kitchen, Bapu stated that it took him 40 years of *sadhana* because he wanted "something that would not fade with time." Forty stands as the number of fulfillment and completion (The Israelites were in the desert for 40 years, and Jesus fasted alone in the desert for 40 days and nights). To do constant spiritual practice alone in the jungle constitutes a desert experience. As a result of these 40 years, which began at quite an early age—for the Supreme never left his heart after his first vision of Lord Krishna—the gift Bapu received from the Divine will not be taken away.

8. The Great Meeting

When I first saw You
I stood amazed, dumbfounded.
When You spoke, it was with my voice and
You gazed at me with my eyes till I died to being other.

—Vishnu Datta—

The Divine is, we could say, the highest abstraction, yet wants to become the greatest concreteness. Heaven adores the Earth. It is, therefore, the Divine delight to act through chosen agents who make tangible and concrete the Divine will.

In November of 1975, Bapu became inwardly aware that he would meet the Lord that night at midnight. He was all day (the 14th day of the month, for he would meet Sadguru Dattatreya on the 15th) in a state of great expectancy—not nervous or apprehensive—for he knew this encounter would fulfill his life and culminate his forty years of arduous spiritual observance.

That night, he brought fruit and flowers and an *asan* (a cloth to sit on) and went to a large rock a short walk from his hut at the ashram. There he sat and waited until midnight. At that hour, the Lord had not appeared, and Bapu wondered if his longing for the Lord's *darshan* (presence) would be fulfilled.

Suddenly, three balls of light from different directions came together to coalesce in the classical form of Lord Dattatreya, with three heads and six arms, each bearing a symbol of divine authority, along with a white cow and four dogs.

Bapu had long wanted to be in the Lord's direct company. Indeed, Bapus' initial burst of spiritual fervor found expression as a boy when he wanted so deeply to see Lord Krishna. Bapu had twice received this great blessing, which, though brief, empowered his life with tremendous longing.

But why would the Lord wish to meet with this unknown renunciate? The Lord, having something to bestow on someone who had proved himself worthy of the greatest of gifts, knew who Bapu was, and knew, therefore, that Bapu would use such a gift wisely, to the greatest benefit, and would give this gift away to everyone who might want it.

Even though this event happened on a specific date on a large rock just a five-minute walk from the ashram, this meeting was bound neither by space or time, but took place in the infinite reaches of Divine love.

9. The Legendary Boon

How did You know exactly what I required?
Your giving took away all my need.
I knew this in the first birth of Your glance.
The gift of gifts was instantaneous with Your breath.

—Vishnu Datta—

As if in an ancient legend, Lord Datta offered Bapu a boon, any wish whatsoever. "What do you want?" the Lord asked.

Whereas in fairy tales boons are usually given to show that desires are often unwise and harmful, this boon was offered by the Supreme to someone who was without desires. The desire came from the Lord, or, more aptly, the desire came from us, from all humanity, from the deep need of our human family to be fulfilled. In this Divine context, the potential of true human beingness is vastly greater than has been represented in any fairy tale.

Who is worthy of being offered a boon from the Lord? Only someone who will not only ask wisely and put to greatest use that which is to be given, but also who has attained a development at least commensurate with the gift to be bestowed. The one who is to be granted a boon, therefore, must be incorruptible as well as wise. Moreover, such a soul would have to be as pure and as potent as the gift itself, lest the inheritance overwhelm the inheritor. Lord Dattatreya knew Bapu was the one.

To the Lord's query, Bapu replied calmly, "I want nothing for myself. I have everything I need."

The Lord's response reiterated His request: "You

must ask for something."

"What could I possibly want, Beloved?" Bapu offered. "You are here!"

Despite such a heartful remark, the Lord was adamant, wanting to give something Divine to His devotee, and with command repeated His question a third time: "You must ask for something."

So it is that Bapu requested something not for himself, but for all humanity, for all of us.

He asked that the Lord give him the most powerful, protected, blessed and integrating spiritual tool possible, a Divine invention that would be especially effective for these challenging times when following the desire for Truth seems so difficult to enact and realize.

10. The Company the Lord Keeps

When I wanted to learn wisdom,
You sent me into the marketplace,
Telling me not to look at the price of things
But into the eyes of the shopkeepers.

—*Vishnu Datta*—

Lord Dattatreya did not reply.

However, Bapu then saw all the *Siddhas*—those perfected souls who guide and guard each of the world's spiritual-religion traditions—surrounding the Lord. Bapu has stated with emphasis, "They all were there, and not one of them was missing."

The *Siddhas*, Bapu realized, were all singing. In unison, they sang out, "*Hari Om Tatsat Jai Guru Datta.*"

Bapu understood that what they were chanting in unison was, indeed, *their* practice, their most cherished and apt way of honoring and being unified with the Supreme. "How old this *Hari Om Tatsat Jai Guru Datta* must be!" Bapu has exclaimed.

Hearing these perfected ones chanting the mantra that they use, Bapu understood that not only was this mantra their *sadhana*, but also that the Lord was giving him the spiritual practice of those so close to the Divine. This, then, was Sadguru's response to his own request that the Lord give him the most powerful and useful, healing and integrating tool possible for human development. What Bapu was too overwhelmed and humble to realize is that this gift was, in the most concentrated form, the inspiration and enactment and completion of his forty years of constant spiritual practice.

11. From the Mouth of the Supreme

The act of true speech
Will not be remembered...
And yet never can be forgotten.
The truth makes hearing and hearer one with the speaker.

—*Vishnu Datta*—

Bapu, wishing to make sure it was this mantra that was Lord's bestowal, asked, "Lord, is this what you mean to give me?"

"Hari Om Tatsat Jai Guru Datta," confirmed the Lord, speaking out the great gift from His own mouth. Then the Guru of Gurus said to Bapu, "Go and give this mantra to everyone who wishes it."

This mantra was given to Bapu in response to his selfless request for something that would most deeply benefit all souls, especially since the spiritual quest is so difficult, fraught with detours and distractions. The Lord had responded, therefore, with the most potent of gifts, the most accurate and palpable weapon, the most relevant and useful of all tools.

Throughout human history, no other spiritual gift, to the author's knowledge, has come directly from the mouth of the Lord. The Vedas were cognized by *rishis* (seers) whose awareness was stationed at the point where Creation is manifesting, and these seers sang out their cognition in verses that became the Vedic hymns. The Torah and Gospel were Divinely inspired writings, without doubt. The Quran was given to the prophet Mohammed (Upon him be peace) over a period of 23 years through the agency of the Angel Gabriel. Certainly Divine incarnations, such as Krishna and

Buddha, have spoken to humanity, and their words stand as the core of the literature of their respective religious traditions. Indeed, every individual may receive guidance and inspiration from the Almighty. And, to be sure, every gift from God is 'direct,' and every authentic agent of God presents only what the Most High endorses. But a spiritual gift for all humanity from the mouth of the Lord of Lords evidently has not been previously recorded.

That this *mahamantra* (great mantra) came so precisely and immediately from the lips of the Divine is the reason that it is so direct in its Divine connection and so saturated with blessings. A frequent word in the vocabulary of those who live at Girnar Sadhana Ashram is 'hotline.' There is something, however ineffable or inexplicable, that is nevertheless actual which—through the agency and blessing of this mantra—comes *directly* from the Lord.

The most stunning moments in the long corridor of human efforts are not always well-reported or even well-understood. Recorded human history celebrates great inventions—from the advent of fire to the electric light, from the wheel to the automobile to the airplane and rocket, from smoke signals to the computer. These innovations have clearly forwarded the potential of our race.

What invention, what innovation could it be that would come from the Source, Course and Goal of all Creation? It is one that would be for every soul, and for the highest degree and dimension of the soul—for fulfillment, for the ultimate conscious possibility, for the greatest ability to serve. This invention that was given to Bapu was a tool that carries the very essence of the Divine nature, a tool powerful enough and integrated enough to bond the Divine nature to our human nature.

---

12. The Ocean in a Bottle

Every raindrop contains a skyful of clouds
And the sea and all its descending rivers.
Every dewed morning could flood the world
　　　　　ten thousand times.
Tell me: What is not water?

　　　　　　　　　　　　　　—Vishnu Datta—

　　　Since the gift of the Supreme was a mantra, we might well inquire into the nature of mantra. Mantra is a word or words of power whose effect is beneficial on all levels of life. Mantra is, we could say, the purest act of poetry. The most concentrated and condensed of poems would be mantra. We could say that life, in a word, is mantra, and mantra, in a word, is life—for a mantra represents the fullness of Creation in a single act of speech. Bapu has said that a mantra is "an ocean in a bottle." The whole universe is, as it were, 'contained' in a word. Entire books have been written about a single mantra.

　　　Mantras are in Sanskrit, the most ancient of languages. A Sanskrit more ancient that what one would study today is likely the "Proto-Indo-European" that linguists theorize is the source of all language. Sanskrit was not invented by human beings, but rather was divinely bestowed. It is called *devanauguri*, divine language. Amazingly, in Sanskrit, a word and what it signifies are vibrationally identical. Someone on the highest level of consciousness could hear a word, say 'library', and know everything about 'library'. That which mantras signify, they are.

　　　What is the meaning of this great *Hari Om Tatsat Jai Guru Datta* mantra? To this frequent question, the most truthful response is that a mantra doesn't 'mean' something. Rather, it 'is' something. A mantra is a name of the Divine. "*Hari Om Tatsat Jai Guru Datta*" is a form of Sadguru," says Bapu. The fullness and completeness of *Hari Om Tatsat Jai Guru Datta* will not be understood except by whoever reaches the culmination of this mantra, which is union with God. "Everything is contained in this mantra," according to Bapu.

Having extended the nature of mantra to the farthest limit of language, still the question of what *Hari Om Tatsat Jai Guru Datta* signifies deserves a solid response, albeit enormously condensed.

Hari: 'Hari' refers to all the love and consciousness that has ever taken form. *Hari* is a name of the Divine. *Hari* refers to the incarnations of the Divine. Rama, Krishna, Buddha, Jesus, Bapu are all *Haris*.

Om: This well-known mantra vibrationally contains the beginning, middle and finale of all of Creation.

Tatsat: 'Tatsat' literally means 'that Truth,' referring to omnipresent Reality, the reality that is everywhere present.

Jai: This mantra is a term of 'victory' or 'glory'.

Guru: While now a dictionary term, the literal meaning of 'gu-ru' is 'darkenss-light'. Thus, a *guru* is someone capable of removing the darkness of ignorance with the light of knowledge. Lord Datta is the Guru of Gurus.

Datta: 'Datta', of course, refers to Lord Dattatreya,
the Datta with three heads (Lords Brahma,
Vishnu and Shiva). But 'Datta' also means 'the
one who gives away all possessions,' or 'the
one who gives all knowledge and wisdom away.'

The *Hari Om Tatsat Jai Guru Datta* mantra far
supersedes the boundary of words, yet our Western
orientation continually wants not only to define, but also to
make a sentence of this *mahamantra*. Even though such an
urge is, from a Vedic understanding, more than simplistic,
nevertheless it deserves an intelligent response. Here is
one possibility: "Glory and victory to the One Giver, that
Omnipresent Truth Who—through the beginning, middle
and end of all Creation—has taken every form of Love
and Consciousness." It should be noted, however, that the
number of 'translations' are virtually unlimited.

And, acknowledging our Western way of understanding,
we might further explicate this mantra in the following way:

Mantra	Divine Qualities	Implement
Hari	Love, Beauty	The Flower
Om	Completeness, Constancy thru time	The Conch
Tatsat	Truth, Reality	The Trident
Jai	Victory, Glory	The Discus
Guru	Wisdom	The Mace
Datta	Abundance, Blessing	The Mala

Hari Om Tatsat Jai Guru Datta, while given in Sanskrit to a great personage in India, is limited by any assumption that it represents Indian knowledge or religion. We do not think of the Law of Gravity is British because its discoverer, Sir Isaac Newton, lived in Great Britain. Rather, it was simply given to Lord Datta's closest friend and lover—who, along with being Indian and deeply in the Vedic tradition, is also a true human being—and was given to be given away to everyone.

13. Giving Away for the Past Thirty Years

The riches you want
Lie, indeed, in the treasure chest.
Open your heart and let the mint be emptied.
Then you, the wealthiest of all beings, will be wealth.

—*Vishnu Datta*—

For the past thirty years, Bapu has been offering the
Hari Om Tatsat Jai Guru Datta mahamantra. He offers it
freely to all, rich and poor, knowledgeable and ignorant, of
every religion.

Usually this takes place at Girnar Sadhana Ashram,
a modest ashram at the foot of Mount Girnar some ten
kilometers east of Junagadh in the Saurastra district of
west-central Gujarat, and just half a mile from the small but
sacred town of Bhavnath. In Rishikesh, about 100 miles
northeast of Delhi, there is another ashram, over the Laxman
Joola footbridge and the last ashram to the left on the banks
of the Ganga. The Trimurti Ganga Ashram is on the Ganges
(Ganga) River, the most sacred of rivers in the Hindu/Vedic
tradition. This ashram is under the guidance of Bapu's
consort, Shri Shailaja Devi (Maiaji). In the hottest months
of the year (May - July), Bapu often visits the Ganges
ashram in Rishikesh.

Bapu does travel around western India, and has
offered many *shabirs* (workshops) in cities such as Bombay,
Ahmadabad, Rajkot, Bhaunagar, Porbandar and Jamnagar.
He twice has come to London and Europe and once, in 1999,
to the United States. However, he has no further plans for
leaving India by plane.

Yet Bapu does travel. At any moment of any day he might be anywhere in the universe. He says, "I do not need a passport." He travels in his *shukshma* (subtle) body… wherever and whenever he wishes, given his inner guidance from Lord Dattatreya. His freedom is solely for the service of others, whoever they are and wherever they might be.

PART II

THE PROMISES

You are here (He points to his heart);
I am there (He points to our heart);
Sadguru is with you 24 hours a day...
Without doubt!

— *Bapu* —

Introduction

This gift—the result of asking the Lord of Lords for the most potent, vital and beneficial instrument for that which most deeply in us longs for fulfillment—holds every truth, every blessing. As Bapu has said, "Everything is there in this mantra."

In our global age, it is imperative that this mantra be utterly unitive. Thus, *Hari Om Tatsat Jai Guru Datta* is offered to all souls, of every color and caste and belief system around the world. It is not more for these kinds of people as opposed to those kinds. No distinctions are drawn.

This mantra is universal yet utterly specific, especially in its healing focus. It is *Hari Om Tatsat Jai Guru Datta* and its promises that get down into the minutiae of our lives, transforming the great and the small. This gift given through Bapu is not for a certain group or kind of people, but for individuals, for each of us specifically. Whatever level we are on, we will be supported and encouraged.

This mantra is able to support every soul exactly where s/he is, yet simultaneously provides the opening door for whatever wants to come into expression.

Hari Om Tatsat Jai Guru Datta is the inspiration prior to religion. It is Veda, Torah, Gospel, Quran. It keeps us growing, from step to step, uniting all paradoxes by simply and profoundly including all aspects and dimensions of the spiritual journey—from beginning to finale—while escaping all definitions, all boundaries, all limitations.

1. Whose Promise?

Who can make an unfailing promise?
One who never fails, never wavers, never falters—
Only that one who has never hesitated, never been flawed,
Can guarantee our light by virtue of having guaranteed
the radiance of all that exists.

—Vishnu Datta—

Whose promises are in this mantra? The One Who from the Alpha to the Omega creates and upholds and fulfills all the worlds is the only One Who could possibly authorize such promises. Such certainty belongs to the Lord of Lords.

No other spiritual gift has actually come from the mouth of the Supreme, the cosmic centrality out of which pours the direct blessings of Lord Dattatreya, the Guru of Gurus. The mantra bears the Lord's name and carries the power and direction of the gaze of God on the spiritual journey of each seeker. By the meaning of the Lord's name, Sadguru Datta ('the one who gives away all possessions') wants to give everything to all who faithfully and sincerely chant this mantra and enjoy the *sahaj dhyan* (Spontaneous Meditation) which follows.

This *mahamantra*, this *siddhamantra* (the mantra of the *Siddhas*), came not from the Vedas, not from some book, not from some saint, not from some cognition—but from the Lord. We don't know of another *mantra* originating in such a divine fashion. It is this directness, this hotline to the highest degree of revelation that so empowers this *mantra* with countless graces and the power to guide, guard and glorify every life.

The first half of the mantra—*Hari Om Tatsat*—has to do with the fullest degree of support and success of our bodily relative nature (creation). The Vedic *rishis* used to chant this mantra—*Hari Om Tatsat*—to gain divine support for all that they needed to accomplish. *Jai Guru Datta* then returns our awareness to Sadguru Datta, and supports our eternal nature (essence). *Jai* means "victory" or "glory." And Guru Datta is the one who can most fully and deeply transform all temporal darkness into the eternal light of knowledge. So within the nature of this mantra we have the fullness of relative life and the fullness of absolute Reality—*purnamidah purnamidam*, as the Vedas say: "All this (Creation) is full and all That (Infinite Reality) is full," thus pointing toward the holographic and indivisible nature of the fullness of life.

Hari Om Tatsat Jai Guru Datta was given to Bapu in response to his selfless request for something that would most deeply benefit all humanity, especially since the spiritual quest is difficult, "...a condition of utter simplicity that demands not less than everything," according to the poet T. S. Eliot. The Lord responded with the most potent gift, the most accurate and powerful weapon, the most relevant and 'user-friendly' tool possible.

Thus it is that all that this *mahamantra* carries comes from the Guru of all gurus. The Lord has spoken in and through this mantra, meaning that the Divine is in this mantra, is sealing the awesome boon via the guarantees in its many promises to whosoever wants to open its gifts. The Supreme has spoken, has directly and lovingly given, and this same voice guarantees the brightness of the future of anyone who enjoys its benefits.

2. Why This Spiritual Tool Now?

Near the poisonous plant, its antidote grows.
The negative sows the seed of the positive,
Today, all is perfectly in order.
Whatever is required appears in the time of clear need.

—*Vishnu Datta*—

Because this mantra was requested and bestowed
in 1975 specifically for this global era of great speed and
unprecedented challenge, chaos, concern and promise—its
blessings are crafted in the *lengua franca* of our modernity,
in the currency we use, in the language that is powerful to
us. Though this mantra is in Sanskrit, its effects are not in
some ancient tongue or out of some ancient era nor do they
require translation, for this mantra, designed for our times,
is helping us here and now in the where and how and why
of our lives. Bapu well understood what kind of challenges
our world would be facing, how vast in significance is this
gateway period. He fully comprehended, better than anyone,
that humanity is entering a watershed crisis, caught between
its high hopes for fulfillment and the dead-end of mere
materiality. This mantra is one of the assurances that the call
to human transformation on our planet will be met.

Only looking back in recognition of having fully
moved through this unprecedented doorway in human history
will we be able to appreciate the gift and its timeliness that
Bapu requested on behalf of all souls. As we penetrate the
veils of ignorance that have kept humanity from its truer
purposes, we will see more and more clearly the dynamic
necessity of why this bestowal took place, and we will

witness that it is the need of our times that brought the antidote for our times. Even a hint of what lies on the other side of that door is brilliant enough to make obvious, based on our own longing for peace and happiness, the fact that the world and its individual souls need real and thorough connection with the Divine. That connection comes through our own self as the concrete expression of the universal essentiality.

3. How Can Such Blessings Be Real and Realized?

Whatever it is we wish to know,
If we look to its source we will see the seed,
The pristine originality of the beginning
Never lost, even until the final fruit.

—Vishnu Datta—

The time for long preparation and meticulous involvement in ritualized particulars in order to attain the purpose of having taken a human body is concluded. Since the inception on Earth of this mantra, the luxury of time has been dwindling, for time itself is being accelerated in this quickening period of phase transition from a denser and less orderly state to a freer and more unified reality.

Life in itself is far from being a complicated affair. What is required has less to do with academic rehearsals and scientific methods of hypothesis and experimentation as it does with the inherent vitality and spirit of being alive. Life does not require PhDs, per se, but does require the qualities of wisdom, honesty, sincerity, strength, faith, courage, unselfishness. What our world lacks is truth and sincerity and corresponding compassion.

In our day, by the grace of God, whoever wants to climb the sacred mountain can do so and will receive guidance for that ascent. Many are the gifts and guides on our planet. The secret is to simply know what we want and, in meeting the gift that we can open (the gift which opens us) to faithfully use this gift and live as best we can. If we follow this deep longing, if we are true to our inner guidance, if we move as our heart quietly dictates—then we will be traveling toward that which every human life has longed for.

With the *Hari Om Tatsat Jai Guru Datta mahamantra*, we merely are beckoned to use it, to sit in Spontaneous Meditation regularly. The frills and gimmicks, the pseudo-spiritual trimmings and tangential efforts have all been mercifully eliminated so that a simple practice can work the simple miracle of life and reveal to us our own true nature and the true nature of all that exists.

The blessings of this mantra are real because *Hari Om Tatsat Jai Guru Datta* bears at least thirteen unique and specific promises, all powerfully essential.

The First Promise:
The State of Meditation Comes Spontaneously

Nature and human nature are one.
There is only one universe, one law.
Everything arises effortlessly from beyond all action.
Why should grace not naturally admit us
*   into our natural home? Hah, there are no gates!*
                                        —*Vishnu Datta*—

In both the distant and recent past, the state of
meditation has represented more the full thrust of spiritual
unfoldment rather than the beginning inspiration. So often
the modality for spiritual aspirants has been to serve a
qualified teacher for a number of years, while moving through
the use of various techniques and practices, until the seeker
was finally initiated into that teacher's main (and often elite)
method of going inward.

With this *mahamantra* given by Lord Datta, the state
of meditation is bestowed without initiation, without deep
instruction, without ritual, without reservation.

The first promise is that, after an individual chants
"Hari Om Tatsat Jai Guru Datta" for 5-10 minutes, the
meditation (*dhyan*) following will be natural, automatic and
spontaneous (*sahaj*). Spontaneous Meditation (*sahaj dhyan*)
happens without effort. It happens each and every time,
whether we chant by ourselves or with a group, whether we
use an audiotape and perhaps offer an invocation or whether
we simply sit and sing it to ourselves in our own home, then
sit with eyes closed.

Hari Om Tatsat Jai Guru Datta is the simplest

in use of all meditative ways. It offers the most receptive possible form of meditation—automatic, spontaneous, natural—in which one needs not remember any practice or methodology but simply sits in the field of promise that comes with this mantra. When Bapu received this mantra from Lord Datta, he was given the finest and most beneficial spiritual tool possible. Therefore, this *mahamantra* is not about technique or methodology. Rather, the coveted state of meditation, sought after by sages and mendicants, comes automatically and without doing. It is called *sahaj dhyan*— Spontaneous Meditation—and it happens simply by our using this tool, chanting this *mahamantra* and then sitting with eyes closed for, say, 20-30 minutes morning and evening.

The mantra *Hari Om Tatsat Jai Guru Datta* is the simplest in use of all mantric practices. Although we are encouraged to bring our sincerity to this practice, in a deep sense, we do nothing and the Lord, through this mantra, does everything, such that the state of meditation, comes automatically—without doing. This great mantra makes the 'not doing' possible.

The Second Promise:
This Gift Is for Everyone

The One I bow to resides brilliantly beyond location.
Every spark has come from this fire.
Not one ember ever goes out.
The Love I love holds every one of us
in Light-filled embrace.

—*Vishnu Datta*—

If you were the Lord, would you not want what you have to offer to be for everyone, for every soul brought into existence? It is so, indeed, with *Hari Om Tatsat Jai Guru Datta.*

The Lord of Lords has given a fulfilled and universal individual a gift meant for everyone. Whether everyone chooses to receive it and use it is, of course, up to each individual's heart and free will. But, regardless, the Supreme has given this unbounded present in a universal way. It is for rich and poor alike, for male and female alike, for those in the East and those in the West, for the young and the old, for those married and those unmarried, for the believers and the non-believers, for the sick and the well, for the accepted and the outcast, for this time and for all times.

The Third Promise:
The Great Helpers Attend Us

The great ones are current. They never leave, only
More and more deeply become. Longing
> *for true community, they willingly invest*
> *in the cause of Truth.*
The coin of their realm is freedom; our freedom
> *means their wealth.*

—*Vishnu Datta*—

When making his request of Lord Datta, suddenly around the form of the Supreme Bapu beheld all the *Siddhas*, at least 84 in number, since there are 84 principle *Siddhas*. These great beings were singing *Hari Om Tatsat Jai Guru Datta*, which is their *sadhana*—the spiritual practice they prefer and how they love to adore the Lord.

This mantra, therefore, bears the promises of no other mantra: that the *Siddhas* will be present to whosoever sincerely chants this *mantra*. If we use this *mahamantra*, we will have the presence of the perfected beings, not just when we chant but in our lives, as well. Drawn by this mantra, they will spontaneously offer the support, the ease and orderliness that naturally emanates from their presence.

Since these *Siddhas* are those great beings who guide and guard each of our planet's spirituo-religious traditions, we will automatically attract those great ones who are most akin to us, whose sphere of influence best matches ours. If, for example, we are Christian, then we will draw to us that influence; if we are Jewish, then we naturally attract the energies deeply linked with that great path. We might draw to ourselves the blessings of the guardian of a path we have either let go of or one which we will come to at some later time in our lives. Regardless, these perfected souls who bear such great and loving responsibility come automatically. We will likely be unaware of their specific presence, yet, without doubt, they will be blessing us.

The Fourth Promise:
Our Protection Is Guaranteed

That which loves naturally protects.
That which is true mirrors and freshly extends the primal order.
Whatever enters the circle of realized harmony
Is either repelled by its mistrust of love
*   or drawn in for long-awaited transformation.*

—Vishnu Datta—

By virtue of the source of this mantra being the purest
and highest revelation, *Hari Om Tatsat Jai Guru Datta* is the
most protecting of all spiritual practices. This great mantra
blesses each *sadhaka* (one who engages in *sadhana*, spiritual
practice) with complete protection on every stratum of
life. The Divine energy of Lord Datta, of Bapu and the 84
principal *Siddhas* permeates *Hari Om Tatsat Jai Guru Datta*.

Just to illustrate its protective power, Bapu once asked
if there was black magic in America. He went on to say that
no negative spirit could withstand the presence of this mantra,
and that any such entity would be forced to leave immediately
by virtue of simply being unable to remain in the field of such
order and love. In another example, a fakir with a certain
power drew people to him and would put them in a trance.
Those who came were asked to leave their wallets, watches
and jewelry outside the fakir's hut, ostensibly so as not to
contaminate the spiritual purity of the fakir with worldly
possessions. But, after the hypnotic trance, they would leave,
forgetting all that they had left behind, and the fakir would
reap his payment. One young man, however, took his wallet
and watch as he left. When stopped and asked by the fakir

how he remembered his valuables, the young man replied simply that he practiced *Hari Om Tatsat Jai Guru Datta.*

In Vedic understanding, the spiritual life is lived through *mantra, tantra* and *yantra. Mantra* is the bestowal of the Divine which, through sound, carries the Divine potency. *Tantra* is spiritual practice, especially that practice which moves beyond the rational into the essential. And *yantra* is a representation in form of the arena of Divine influence. In the Vedic pantheon, every Law of Nature is embodied, and each embodiment has his or her own arena of influence and, therefore, his or her own *yantra.* To view the Datta Yantra, which represents Bhagawan Dattatreya's gift and energy is to behold the most complete and intricate of all the *yantras* (sacred forms). Therefore, the field of orderliness, generated through Lord Dattatreya and depicted in His *yantra,* is the most protective possible.

The Datta Yantra represents the field of orderliness that surrounds each *sadhaka* who uses *the Hari Om Tatsat Jai Guru Datta mahamantra.* That orderliness surrounds and permeates whoever—whether an individual or a group—chants this mantra and sits immediately afterwards in meditation. This great organizing power affects the families, homes and places of employment of anyone who uses this *mahamantra* in his or her *sadhana.*

The Fifth Promise:
Maturity Comes through Integration

I yearn to thrive inseparable from fullness,
Beyond the myriad distances of opposites.
The fire and the water made such love
That both died into me who lives for and in the flow of light.
—Vishnu Datta—

Hari Om Tatsat Jai Guru Datta supports each of us exactly where we are. It gives blessings on every level of our lives. Why? Because this *mantra* is *sahaj*, is natural, is life itself. It brings about spiritual development in a totally organic and authentic way, without emphasizing one arena of growth over another. Rather, all venues of maturity are stimulated, each in its own manner and flow, each in its own specialty and in its harmony with all other inputs into our moment-by-moment being as we spontaneously unfold.

Our proclivity for the five senses and the numberless sense objects keeps our attention mainly oriented toward those developments we can see. However, perhaps the greatest spiritual quality we, if we are interested in maturity, could want is *integration*. Integration, if it were, say, a film star, would have a small but sincere and devoted following whose numbers were lower than all other film stars, except perhaps those fans of Humility. Were Integration a sports celebrity, s/he would spent the vast majority of time on the bench. Yet integration represents true spiritual maturation.

Integration is little understood and appreciated, because it involves a dying. Blue and Yellow both lose their individual identities in their integration as Green. If we have experience 'X' and then another experience 'Y', integrating these two experiences means coming to a state in which they are both present, but not as before. They become 'XY', which means not just 'X' and not just 'Y'. We have both together, but neither individually, and in that sense there may seem to be less 'X' and less 'Y'. Yet the actuality is that both 'X' and 'Y' are significantly stronger as 'XY'.

The wise understand that far more useful and beneficial than having many experiences is being able to integrate the experiences we do have. Someone who has a hundred experiences and integrates only a few is less developed and less mature than someone who has ten experiences and integrates them all.

Bapu, for example, is the most integrated of human beings. He is like a diamond whose facets are so numerous that they virtually disappear into the smoothness of a sphere. Other great souls, with maybe a dozen well-developed facets, may seem more fascinating and we might feel that they possess a greater luster. However, when a quality is integrated, it can be truly used, and can be more deeply used the more deeply integrated it is into our own natural state of being.

The Sixth Promise:
Energy Is Released and
Channeled in the Body

We fear the world; we fear creation...
Until the radiance of firstness enters us—
Limbs, head and heart---so we know we are the leaves,
*   the rivers and rain, the mountains, the moon and stars.*
See! How could it have ever been otherwise?

—Vishnu Datta—

Hari Om Tatsat Jai Guru Datta is definitely directed to release the body's own spiritual energies. Known in the Vedic tradition as *kundalini shakti*, our natural spiritual energy lies dormant at the base of the spine—until it is awakened. *Shakti* means 'power,' and *Kundalini* refers to a '*kundal*', a circular earring, signifying the circle of completion that this primal energy wants to make in our bodies by moving through all the energy centers, called *chakras*.

Chakra means 'wheel'. When opened, each *chakra* will begin to spin. The *chakras* are subtle gathering points along the spine which store the impressions of the difficult experiences we have taken on. As a given *chakra* turns, its gathering speed spins away the dust and debris of the overwhelming impressions that we have stored in our nervous systems. Everything is turning—day and night, our Earth and its moon, our solar system. When we start consciously turning, we start consciously participating in the nature of Creation.

Each *chakra* is associated with an arena of limited human identification which, functionally, keeps our attention identified with an agenda that cannot possibly bring happiness.   The energy of each *chakra* is also associated with a color. Experiences in meditation may comment, via color and/or location of bodily sensations, which *chakra* is being purified. While books have been written about the intricacies of the *chakra* system, the following delineations will be sufficient for the purposes of this book.

Number	Name	Location	Issue	Color
First	*Muladhara*	Base of the spine	Security	Red
Second	*Manipura*	Just below the navel	Pleasure & Esteem	Orange
Third	*Swadishtana*	The solar plexus	Power & Control	Yellow
Fourth	*Anahata*	The heart	Objectivity	Green
Fifth	*Vishuddhi*	The throat	Expression, Command	Blue
Sixth	*Agya*	Between the brows	Clarity, pure perception	Indigo
Seventh	*Sahaswara*	Crown of the head	Fullness of life	Violet/White

The *Hari Om Tatsat Jai Guru Datta mahamantra* brings such primal energy toward expression and completion, so that in us liberation becomes actual and not merely mythological or ideational. We do not want to make a mood of spirituality; rather, we want to actually wake up—in our minds and in our hearts, but also in our bodies, as well as in our soul. We each long for tangible experiential results and not just theoretical or theological understandings.

When the *kundalini* energy penetrates a given *chakra*, the issues of that arena release their relational materials and we experience perhaps intense corresponding purification. When the *shakti* starts to penetrate a *chakra*, its wheel starts to spin off the debris of any limiting agendas, a process that accelerates as the speed of the spin increases. The *chakras* can be stimulated well before their actual opening, such that the process of purification can begin early on. *Hari Om Tatsat Jai Guru Datta* directly stimulates the rise of the *shakti,* whose coursing through the nervous system moves our relationship to life well beyond theory. The completion of the *kundalini shakti*—the clear circuit of internal energy that is the gift of all the chakras having been penetrated and cleansed by the *shakti*—means real aliveness. It is vitally important that this *mahamantra* does not merely stimulate the primal *kundalini* power, but that it also governs it, constantly integrating it so that this power, which is identical to the power of Creation, works in and with us and not against us, which is to say that we will not be overcome by this power, but empowered by it.

The first part of the mantra—*Hari Om Tatsat*—stimulates the *Ida,* the moon channel beginning on the left side of the spinal column, while the second part—*Jai Guru Datta*—stimulates the *Pingala,* the sun channel originating on the right side of the spinal cord. Between these two nerves is the hair-fine *sushumna* through which the *kundalini shakti* rises when the inner development of the *sadhaka* is ready for the lessons and clearing that each of the *chakras* represents. The reward is growing bliss, integrity and spiritual maturity.

The development of the *chakras* is independent of spiritual states—such as awakening, realization, liberation and enlightenment. As the *chakras* open, more vitality and depth, more fluidity and fearlessness move through us. To have the *chakra* system open and functioning is to have all life impulses available. Rather than equivalent to spiritual states, the *chakras* are more about becoming a true human being, a completely alive individual.

In many traditions, this *shakti* is not spoken of. These

paths on this matter are hushed because of the dangers so often encountered with this primal urge of life—for the power, purification, freedom and life force of this energy have, without the integrating safeguards of this mantra, been striking and even harrowing, for the effects in the body of the *shakti* are utterly unique and, therefore, this primal power makes a pioneer out of every soul. Other teachings put specific attention on the *chakras* and offer specific practices to ignite and raise the *shakti*. Such spiritual practices which directly try to focus on the *kundalini shakti* take chances if they are based on book knowledge or on the experience of a realized teacher who may not be well-enough acquainted with not only the intricacies of the *shakti* but also the larger arenas of the s*hakti's* influence. What is important here with regard to *Hari Om Tatsat Jai Guru Datta* is that this mantra is so protective and deeply integrating as to prevent the commonly feared dangers about this mysterious but natural energy being expressed. It is not just the stimulation and expression of the *kundalini shakti* that is the blessing of this *mahamantra*, but also the integration of this spiritual energy. Thus, safety is always present. It should be mentioned that, when this energy pierces the nexus points of congealed limiting beliefs, the process can be challenging. With this mantra, this inherently challenging process is 'governed' so as to not become overwhelming.

　　　Hari Om Tatsat Jai Guru Datta, therefore, represents not only the fullness found in the development of consciousness, but also the longing to be a true human being. Higher states of consciousness are to bring closer and closer identification of who we really are with the very nature of Reality—until unity is achieved, a motion of expansiveness, of Heaven. The *kundalini shakti* is to root us incarnationally in our bodies, a motion of depth, of Earth. Some religions are directed toward Paradise, while others aim at the blessings of our Mother Earth. These two 'directions'—the upward orientation and the downward orientation—have over the centuries developed into enemies. The *Hari Om Tatsat Jai Guru Datta mahamantra* leaves nothing out, for it unites all limitations and differences, thus fulfilling both primal spiritual orientations—both in terms of consciousness and in terms of human beingness. Thus is this mantra a vehicle for both inner and outer peace.

The Seventh Promise:
Everything We Require Comes to Us

When we wait without expectation, all things come to us.
It is so because our cup needs filling.
Neither ignoring nor squandering what we receive,
We become patience, flowing over our rims like a fountain.

—Vishnu Datta—

Imagine the comfort of living life in the awareness
that every possible experience that we each uniquely
need will come to us naturally and automatically without
our having to 'make it happen.' To use this *mahamantra*
regularly means that we are drawing to ourselves all our
necessary experiences. Every next step will naturally and
automatically present itself to the *sadhaka*, wherever he or
she lives. With continued use of *Hari Om Tatsat Jai Guru
Datta*, all the unique experiences we each require for our
fulfillment will spontaneously be ushered to us, so that
life will be *sahaj* and we will move optimumly toward the
ultimate state of *sahaj yoga*.

Sahaj Yoga is the motion of life naturally and
spontaneously toward union with Reality. '*Yoga*' means
'union with our own eternal nature.' *Sahaj Yoga* walks
the fine line between personal and impersonal, being
simultaneously both and beyond both. This *Sahaj Yoga*
brings in an organic fashion all the experiences each of us
requires. Even though its purpose and goal is to lead us
beyond experience to the Source of all experiences, still each
of us requires unique inner and outer events personal only
to us that will bring the realizations and faith to forward our

spiritual growth. We may sees visions—of God, of deities, of sages, of our own guru—or enjoy various communications filled with knowledge, or feel exhilarated and permeated by the *kundalini shakti*. Whatever experiences we have, each is necessary to our growth in spirit.

Moreover, the *sahaj* nature of this mantra means that it leads to the summit of spiritual development. Even *yogis* in *nirvikalpa samadhi* (unbroken state of Reality), still long for *sahaj yoga*, the constant contact with the ubiquitous Source of Life, that natural state of living the Truth in all its forms and expressions, accepting everything and everyone as the expression of Divine Intelligence.

The Eighth Promise:
All Yogas Are Contained in This Mantra

The gift of a seed is a tree.
The gift of a tree is a forest.
The gift of a forest is a habitat for living.
Take me to the treasury of life that holds all presents.

—Vishnu Datta—

Hari Om Tatsat Jai Guru Datta is a spiritual
practice of chant, meditation and *jaapa* that is a *yoga*
exactly mirroring the way life operates, that is as natural as
nature, that fluidly escapes all categories and artificialities.
It is life itself gifting us in the most intimate and unitive
ways possible.

The regular practice of this mantra is termed *Sahaj
Yoga.* What that means is, via this mantra, that all the
yogas—*karma* (the *yoga* of selfless action), *hatha* (the *yoga*
of force, of physical postures), *bhakti* (the *yoga* of devotion),
jyana (the *yoga* of discrimination and knowledge), *kriya* (the
yoga of working with subtle internal energies), *laya* (the *yoga*
of one moment changing into another), to name just the main
yogic paths.—will spontaneously announce themselves in
the body and awareness of the seeker who progresses in this
inclusive way. Every *asana* (posture), *pranayama* (flow of
breath), teacher, book and initiation will spontaneously find
the student of this mantra. There is no longer the need to go
looking for the next step of our spiritual journey.

Bapu has said that life can hold all the *yogas*, not just
that single stream for which we would each have the greatest
proclivity. Rather, he says, the many *yogas* are like cars on a

train, and that we can enjoy and attain them all, enjoying the entire train rather than being confined to a single car.

Nothing is denied the one who faithfully moves in the blessings of Sadguru Dattatreya.

The Ninth Promise:
Receiving Answers Inside

What is greater than the greatest
Is no different from what is smaller than the smallest.
To move deeper is to move higher.
Wherever the truth of love takes us, our vista is both wider and
more focused: Love's universe on a pinpoint.

—Vishnu Datta—

To grow maturely in the way of the fullness of life is
to be freer to be ourselves, to be natural and complete human
beings. Therefore, our inner guidance develops, increases
and grows clearer with this mantra, for our inner 'voice' is
Sadguru within us. The inner *guru* comes alive, and we trust
this natural intelligence, which is our own, more and more.

Moreover, if we have questions, we are invited to ask
in meditation and receive answers. Indeed, Bapu encourages
us to ask in meditation, to get our own answers from inside,
responses which are far fuller and better, more relevant and
more lasting than what even he could verbally offer. To ask
in meditation means that, prior to *sahaj dhyan*, we simply
state our request, and then let the Lord of Spontaneous
Meditation respond whenever and however is best.

Bapu does not tell us what to do, except perhaps
in emergencies, for he does not interfere in our free will.
His guidance is subtle, is given in hints and never attracts
attention to himself. In the same way, the Lord of Lords
through this mantra works in us.

The Tenth Promise:
There Are No Rules

Those who thirst and would steal water from others
Require that love rules them with rules.
But the fertile fields of the Most High
Are flooded.

—*Vishnu Datta*—

This *mahamantra* supports us in the daily workings of our lives. It meets our individual needs and callings, and its blessings come directly. Because of the universality of the gift of *Hari Om Tatsat Jai Guru Datta*, this mantra bears no confinement—not of person or of ritual or of practice (except that practice is required if we want to grow in its promises... and the more regular our use, the more constant and deep our development). Though *Hari Om Tatsat Jai Guru Datta* has grown out of a Vedic cultural milieu, the only thing required of this spiritual tool is our using it.

Sadguru Datta has been known to appear in physical form. Reports of such encounters usually have the Lord posing as a madman or a farmer, an appearance not only confounding expectations but also demanding a deeper look than the physical eye can offer. With the Lord, author of both the structure (law) and essence (process) of all Creation, there are no givens, no proprieties, no rules. The Lord simply wants our authentic freedom born of conscious contact with our lasting nature.

In that way, our freedom naturally grows with this mantra—not in the way of license, but in all the ways of beauty, joy, love and harmony—both individually and relationally.

The Eleventh Promise:
We Become Ourselves

Whenever it was that I realized
No one else's finger could point my way and
No other tongue could describe the terrain of my going,
I found the map of guidance had been written indelibly
*   on the parchment of my heart, a map only I could trust.*
                                        —Vishnu Datta—

The nature of the ego is to try to make itself the sole power of its universe, and to make other egos bow to its authority. Hence, greed, control and even violence are rampant on every level—from personal to communal to international—in our modern world.

The magnitude and magnanimity of this *mahamanta* is the very generosity of the Lord Who has created all souls and loves every being. Thus, we are guided and inspired by this Divine gift to become exactly who we—in our utter uniqueness and our complete universality—have been designed to be. We are not being groomed to be or think or dress or act like anyone else, but are released into our own energy to enact what our nervous system was made to support. That service—that *dharma*, that sacred offering of ourselves in the duties we are best suited to offer—is exactly what this *sadhana* is revealing in us.

Hari Om Tatsat Jai Guru Datta supports us exactly where we are—in all our moods and changes and repositionings—so that we are always on course, our life heading for the most abundant of destinations.

The Twelfth Promise:
This Mantra Constitutes a Complete Practice

The map to vastness
Has countless turns to one who is counting.
To one with simple faith,
The next step is the secret to the whole journey.

—Vishnu Datta—

One of the main themes regarding the uniqueness of this mantra is the holistic nature of its benefits—both absolute and relative, both impersonal and personal, both detailed and vast in its unfathomable intelligence.

Any spiritual gift that proposes to qualify as a complete practice must be able to guide aspirants to the limit of human potential. Many are the incidents in which saints visiting Bapu at Girnar Sadhana Ashram tell him that they are at a plateau in their sadhana and ask what to do. "Here," says Bapu, "take this mantra, *Hari Om Tatsat Jai Guru Datta.*" In this gesture, he is offering them all he has, for this mantra is the synthesis, as in the extreme distillation of a homeopathic remedy, of Bapu's 40-year *sadhana*, a *sadhana* which made him a master of *sadhana*. Thus, this *mahamantra*, while not withheld from beginner, does not fail to continue to lead the leaders, experts and aficionados.

Also required for a 'complete practice' is that the guide to such a gift resides and is integrated at the apex of human development. Since the guru of this practice is Sadguru Datta, such a qualification is satisfied to the fullest. Then, too, Bapu is the most integrated of human beings, is one with the Guru of gurus, and his grace floods through this *mahamantra*. Only direct experience of this mantra, however, can verify such an assertion.

Another requirement of a complete practice is the singularity of the gift. *Hari Om Tatsat Jai Guru Datta* is the only mantra that Bapu offers those who come for guidance. It is not, as with many spiritual lineages, that one does an initial practice and then, after so many years, receives the main or secret practice.

This mantra is, therefore, utterly complete. Everything will find us. It blesses us both relatively—for we won't grow spiritually if we cannot be sustained in our body, for example, or if our work is too taxing—and absolutely (with Self-Realization, if we simply persist with faith and surrender). This mantra is enormously practical at the same time as it is fully spiritual and ultimately unites all dualistic positionings.

By bringing internally and externally all the experiences we require in our unique journey, this mantra proves itself. It is imperative that God 'prove' His/Her divinity in us as we each need to receive this reality. As quantum physics states, every particle contains the whole of Creation. Therefore, though paradoxically, we are each the center of the universe and the universe needs to reveal itself in terms that we each value and can understand. Thus, this mantra is fully personal, while directing us gently and profoundly beyond the personal/impersonal duality.

Which leads us to another important aspect of *Hari Om Tatsat Jai Guru Datta*. With many spiritual practices, the practitioner grows more and more even and subdued, shunning society and his/her duties in the world. Bapu, who followed the renunciate path for 40 years of total dedication, and Mataji are paragons of human development. This mantra creates in us a greater evenness of temperament and an authentic detachment that saves us from unnecessary suffering. Yet at the same time we grow more capable in the world and more passionate—caring more, not less, more able to express our own inner and outer nature. Such passion plus the great development of consciousness make us true human beings.

Several Magnificent Bonuses

The Potential for Healing Is Unlimited

Many long to quench the thirst of others
Yet find holes in their waterskins.
The opening of a falls in the chest
Floods all need for containers.

—Vishnu Datta—

Given the nature of life as an opportunity to move through layer upon layer of limited assumptions toward a state of freedom beyond assumptions, we will best understand our human situation as one that continually requires healing. Every step of our journey engenders, or is the result of, healing. Healing results from any experience which moves one state of appreciation to the next.

Our current western medical mentality teaches us to be suspicious of any healing modalities not associated with licensed academic programs. While no specific healing claims are made on behalf of the *Hari Om Tatsat Jai Guru Datta* mantra, we can recognize that the Lord of Lords must be the supreme healer. This, after all, is His/Her mantra. Using this mantra calls on the infinite power and potentiality for healing—on every level of our being, from gross to subtle. Bapu has said, "Everything that has gone in must come out." In this way we come to purity and peace.

Perhaps the best way to speak of this promise is a dream, given to the author. Blue ambulances, standing for various spiritual paths, are driving through the streets. Some are cruising the main boulevards. Others, though fewer, are driving up and down the main cross streets. Fewer still are moving along the side streets. One, however, is able to not only drive on all these passageways, but also comes down the alleys and will even find someone on the 17th floor! This ambulance represents the precise and minute healing capacity of this *Hari Om Tatsat Jai Guru Datta mahamanta.*

Life presents itself as energy, which manifests in waves, in patterns. From the expansion and contraction of the universe to day and night, from biorhythms to the beating of hearts—all of Creation is vibration. Each being, each creation, has a vibrational nature, whose energy encodes the unique form which each specific intelligence takes. Since life is layered, each stratum has its own energy band, some bands employing slower and more obvious wavelengths, while others are more rapid, subtle and essential. Most spiritual gifts deal with the slower, more expressed energies. *Hari Om Tatsat Jai Guru Datta,* the most complete and intelligent of all mantras, works on all our energy bands—from the most obvious to the most refined and subtle. Healing, therefore, can be complete via this *mahamantra,* whose power for peace and purity will address every level of our functioning, no matter how hidden or nuanced.

We require healing to move in our personal growth. However, not all our personal ailments must be totally remedied in order for the river of our universal growth to move toward the sea. Thus, our relationship with all issues of healing retains the inherent mystery of life—all that happens to us comes to us by grace rather than through our conscious will and actions. Coming to this mantra with faith and sincerity is entering the nurturing and healing grace of the Supreme, such that the Divine works more and more through us as we continue to grow from wholeness to greater wholeness.

Because this mantra is about our journey to fulfillment, all the healing required for our fulfillment will come to us—likely in surprising ways and unpredictable means.

Bapus' Grace

Inside my inmost garden is that sky
Which makes what we call 'sky' seem smaller than a seed.
Not the first one to be planted in this expanse,
I follow the scent of the freshest and most ancient of roses.

—*Vishnu Datta*—

Although the humblest of souls, without doubt Bapu concretely conducts the blessings of the Supreme. The Divine grace requires transfer points, much the same way a tree trunk branches into limbs, an electric current needs a transformer between the power station and the individual home, or we must fly through Frankfurt or Singapore on our way to Bombay. Bapus' manifold ways of giving almost never call attention to himself, for he needs no acknowledgement.

While scientific instruments will not be able to record or measure this dimension of beauty, clearly the grace of Bapu, while not a promise of this Divine boon, is a reality of direct blessing for those drawn to this mantra. Indeed, Bapu has said that, though this is his last lifetime on Earth, he "will not rest" until all those who have come to this *Hari Om Tatsat Jai Guru Datta mahamantra* are established in the complete state of freedom. Although not included as a promise spoken by Sadguru Dattatreya, this promise comes from Bapu's mouth and constitutes as deep a guarantee.

This Gift Can Be Given to Others

I have no powers.
No magic, no wonders are worked through me.
For only one thing do I want—
That all that I receive I can give away.

—Vishnu Datta—

Because this mantra was given for the benefit of every soul, because it comes to all freely and without reservation, and because there is no organizational hierarchy in charge of meting out or adjudicating its benefits, there is no regulation about sharing this gift with others. Indeed, Bapu encourages us to give it away. We can, therefore, directly benefit the evolutionary progress of our friends and anyone we meet by sharing this easy- to-pronounce, easy-to-use gift that actually came from the mouth of the Supreme. We don't need to be well-educated or to have taken some teacher-training course. After chanting this mantra aloud for 5-10 minutes and then closing our eyes, there is nothing to do and the process moves by itself very experientially. The Lord does it all. If someone needs more knowledge or has questions, this book will serve them well.

PART III

A HANDFUL OF CLARITIES

"Do you know what meditation is?"

— *Bapu* —

*(Asking a 25-year practitioner of meditation,
who could only answer, "I'm not sure.")*

Introduction

Life is everywhere, in everything from the largest of the large to the smallest of the small. Indeed, we have before us a metaphor of human life in every tree and plant. Many spiritual traditions see all of life as a tree. Just as rivers receive the branches of many creeks, veins branch out into capillaries, neurons branch out into dendrites and the arm branches out into the fingers of the hand, the principle of the many—limbs, branches and twigs—being expressed out of the one trunk is concrete and obvious. The entire organism is moving toward the light. Yet this display totally depends on what is unseen. It is the root that, below ground and unavailable to our five senses, determines the life and greatness of all that we sensually call a tree. How apt that a tree's root system usually spreads out underground the same distance as its canopy extends above ground

In a tree, the whole story of our journey is directly before us...and so simple: We are growing out of what is unseen, expressing both unity and diversity, to the one light that gives life to every living thing—a metaphor that may be without impact to those who have no idea how to contact the root of their being.

A Practical Case for Meditation

If you are not looking, why have you read this far?
If you are looking, why have you not yet found the secret?
Sleep is for waking, waking for becoming, becoming for being.
You are the paradox beyond paradise.

—Vishnu Datta—

Even though our full humanity is a natural state—
indeed, is our birthright—we do need a way, a path, a proven
motion into our true nature. Our root, as the root of any plant,
is unseen—yet utterly real and requires water. Actually, it does
not require water if we want merely to survive, to breathe and
move our limbs, to be the product of a single birth. But if we
wish to be fully alive, then our rebirth will come only to the
extent that we do water the root of our very being.

Taking our attention inward, to our root, is the process
of meditation. Meditation is a repeatable (though every
meditation is unique) way of quieting and empowering the
mind, while simultaneously giving great ease to the body.

It is commonly understood that we humans use
but a fraction, about $1/10^{th}$, of our mental potential. Albert
Einstein felt he used 20%. Likely, we have judged some of
our associates as one-percenters, and honesty would likely
have us admitting that we have on occasion behaved that
way ourselves. Can we really hope to use 100%? Full
potential would seem a natural condition, since such a
potential is within each of us. Yet human history and our own
sojourn thus far seem all too often to point to an opposite
conclusion—that tapping into our full potential would be
rather 'superhuman'.

The premise of this handbook not only assumes that full human development and expression is precisely what life is asking of us—and constitutes 'why' we have taken a precious human body—but also provides a way to accomplish this universal goal.

Why meditation? Here, a concrete physiological approach may outperform all the grand and often esoteric rationales proposed throughout the ages, for meditation is the most ancient of ways into our inmost domain. The reason we humans use a humbling 10% of our potential is that we get only that much daily rest, which comes through sleep. In deep sleep, we receive just an 8-10% rest. That 10% rest addresses solely our fatigue, which is sleep's purpose: to refresh us from daily fatigue. For example, imagine a limp neuron restored to elasticity, strength and readiness after a good night's repose. But what about twisted neurons or, worse, neurons that have become crushed or knotted? We all know we have ingested experiences of loss, fear and pain far denser and more difficult than fatigue. To "straighten out" such difficulties requires a far deeper and fuller rest. Which is what meditation offers.

As such rest penetrates our psyches, our hearts and our physical bodies, our lives become more expressive, more intelligent and alert, more resilient and focused, freer and more creative…to name but a smattering of important personal qualities that improve though meditation. As a result, our spirit is strengthened and readied for the many mysteries of what it means to be alive.

Given the dozens or even hundreds of meditation methodologies and practices, the meditation described in this book is important because, regardless of method or technique, there still remains the sneaky question: How do I meditate? That query is answered by Spontaneous Meditation—not a method or technique, not even a meditation, but rather the state of meditation that happens naturally, automatically, spontaneously.

A Trinity of Misconceptions

Meditation Is Not
Making the Mind Blank

Seeing is the first act of any art.
see, the object must be held still.
When we look steadfastly, the object falls away
And we stand in the light of our seeing.

—Vishnu Datta—

If the popular understanding about meditation were encapsulated, it would read: "Meditation is about making the mind a blank." Reducing such a profound state of affairs to a soundbite creates a caricature opposite to the Divine purpose of such a gift.

The state of meditation is dynamic, is an ever-growing relationship to infinite consciousness. The purpose of meditation is not to withdraw from life, but rather to engage with our lives in deeper and wider and more focused contexts, such that we gain in our mental, emotional and spiritual capacities, both quantitatively and qualitatively.

That the mind enters into a state beyond all thought is a distinct possibility in meditation, yet such a state, far from the mind going 'blank', constitutes the most fulfilling and fascinating experience we humans can have. Finally, meditation is not a trance. Rather, our limited ego—and its separate state of identification with objects of experience—is the trance.

An integrated understanding of meditation recognizes that thoughts are a part of meditation, that they are arising naturally, that they represent the purification process. Thus, we come to see that meditation is less about not having thoughts as it is not being attached to the rising and falling of the thoughts that one is naturally having. It is a fairly common experience with *sahaj dhyan* (Spontaneous Meditation) following the *dhun* (chanting) of the *Hari Om Tatsat Jai Guru Datta* mantra that the meditator will experience an inner sense of peace and noticeable stability even though the mind is still producing a constant stream.

The Meditative Engine Has Two Pistons

Down into loam I plunge my blade—
So easy when the soil is wet, dark, aerated.
But to make a hole, I have to shovel out what I've loosened.
Little ins and outs create the great depth.

—Vishnu Datta—

Any sincere meditator needs to clearly comprehend that meditation has two motions: peace and purification. These two pistons propel the engine of meditation and all spiritual growth. Peace is an inward stroke leading to rest, and purification is an outer stroke, the result of healing.

Peace, being ease and simplicity, is a state we all enjoy and favor. Purification, on the other hand, is a state whose discomforts we usually want to avoid. It represents a significant maturity on the part of a meditator to welcome purification as well as peace. Both are necessary, and the spiritual engine will not move without the presence of both.

Every Meditation Is the Best

I have held so many bouquets of opinion.
None lasted long enough to present. Cut flowers wilt.
Now I give my heart, instead.
These petals hold the dew in the fragrance of the moment.

—Vishnu Datta—

While it is natural to prefer peaceful meditations over challenging meditations, the wisdom of experience speaks clearly: Every meditation is the best that could have occurred at that time and under the current specific conditions. Therefore, all judgments about meditations—that morning meditations are better (or worse) than evening meditations, or that today's meditation was deeper than yesterday's— are erroneous, no matter how they may seem to prove themselves. If we judge our meditations subjectively, then we erect an inner wall. Behind that wall we will subtly resist much of what is helpful to us whenever the taste is less than sweet. Our non-judgment of our meditations is paramount, if we wish to surrender to the Divine, such that "Thy will, not mine, be done."

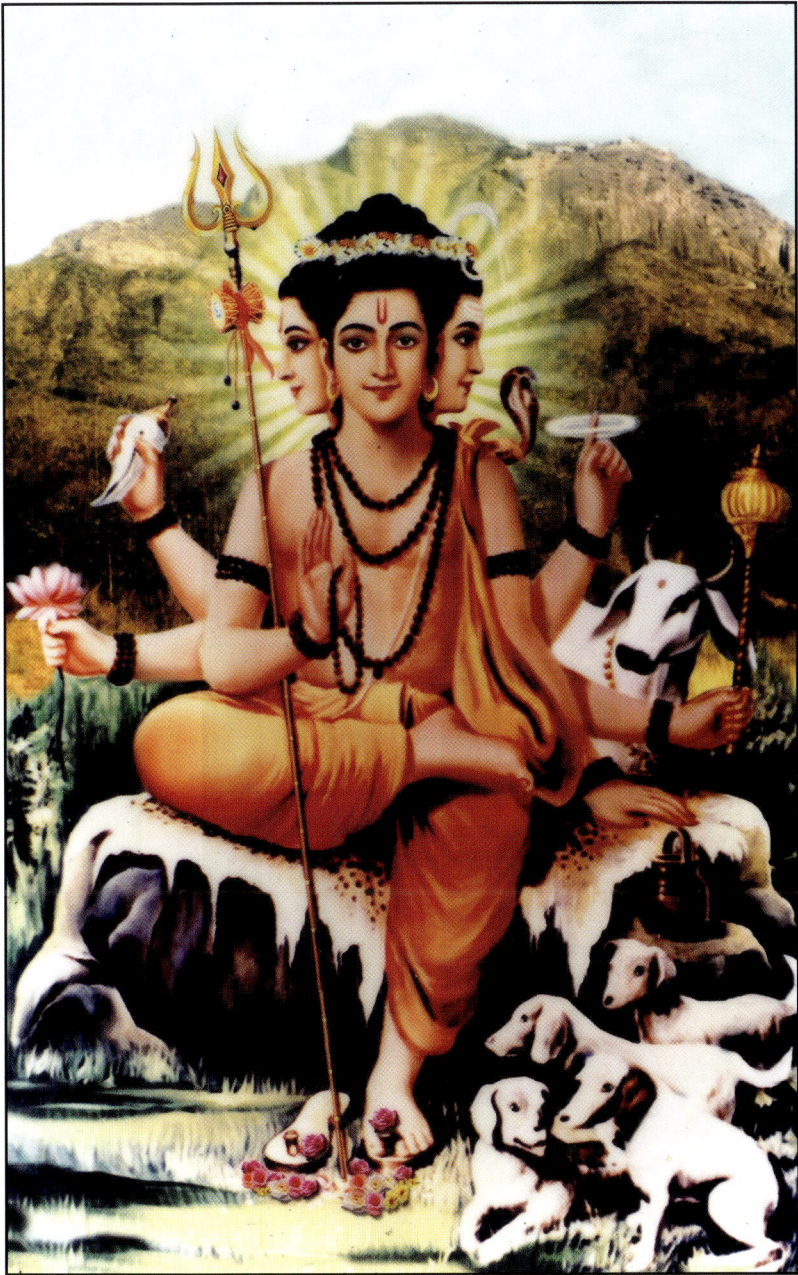

Lord Dattatreya

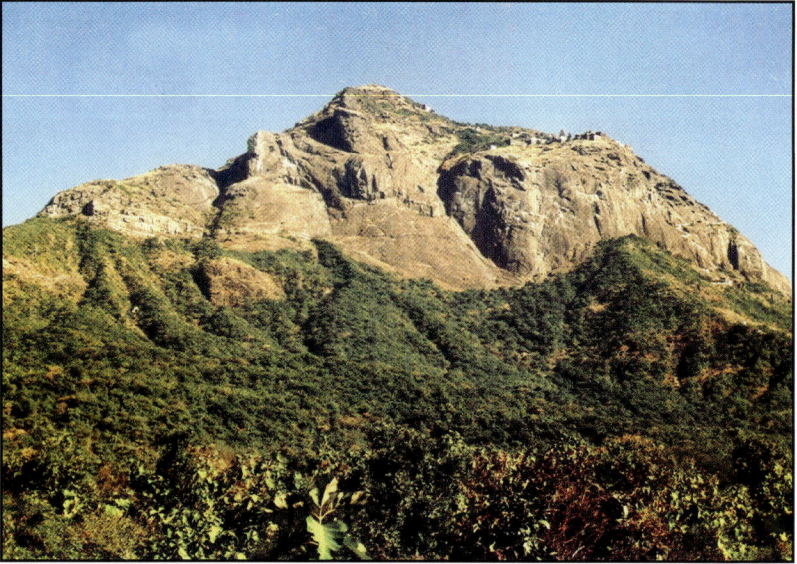

Mount Girnar

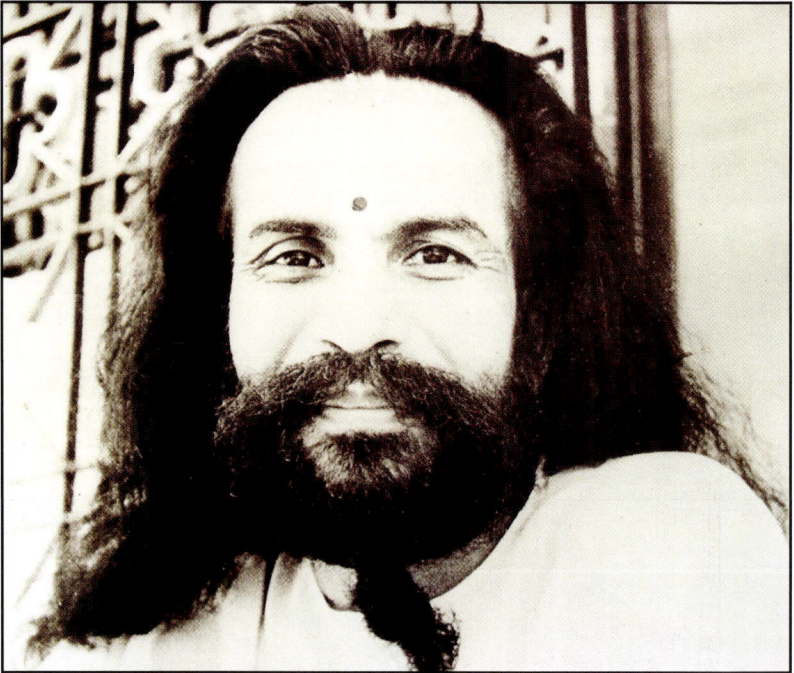

Shri Punitachariji Maharaj (Bapu) 1984

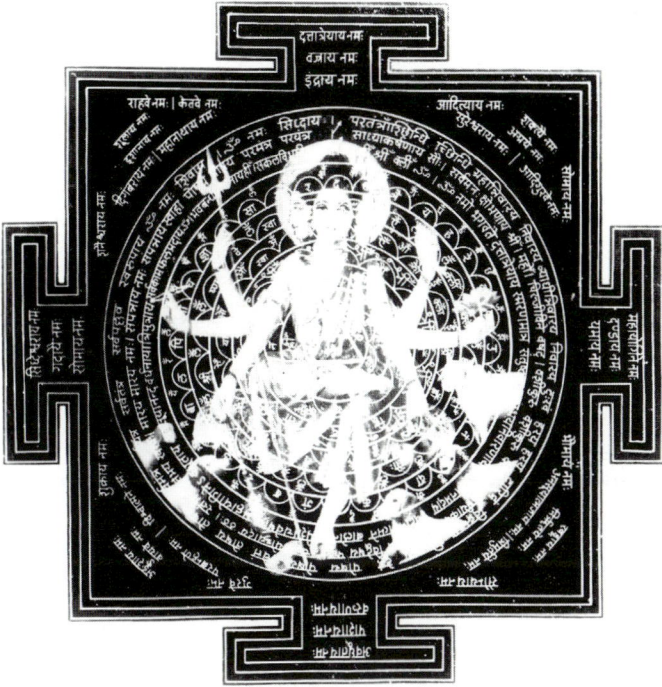

The Datta Yantra

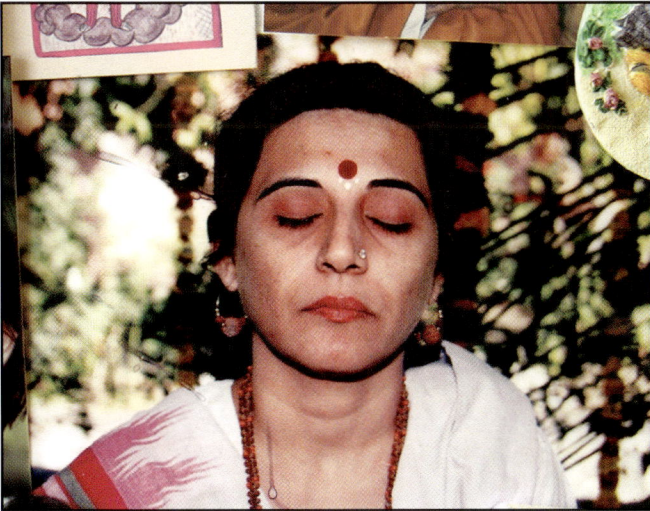

Guru Ma Shailija Devi (Maiaji)

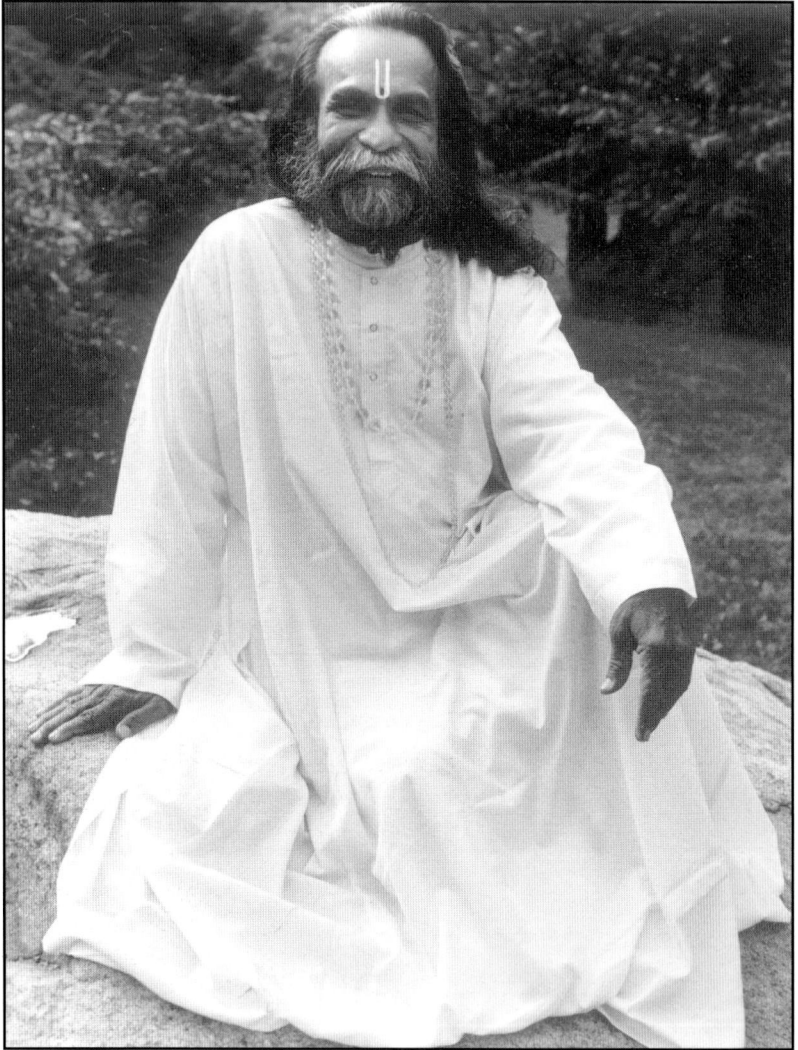

Bapu in America 1999

photo by monika merva

Prime Clarifications

How Far Can This Gift Be Opened?

The present I long for I cannot quite describe.
And so I keep tearing off the wrapping...
Box after box until the boxes end.
Whatever is left is what I have asked for with my every breath.
—*Vishnu Datta*—

This *mahamantra*, originating from the lips of the
Lord, is unlimited in its capacity to give. What, then, is
possible for human beings to receive?

Life is layered, like our nervous systems, like an
onion, like the Grand Canyon. Each layer, when penetrated,
reveals a wider and more vivid outlook, though not denying
the views of all previous strata. We human beings enjoy at
least several states of consciousness: We sleep; we dream; we
are in some state of waking. Each of these states is obviously
quite different from the other two and seems complete in
itself. Each of these states—*sleeping, dreaming* and *waking-*
-are necessary to human life and its functioning. There are
definitely other states of consciousness of which we are
capable. These other states are also necessary—if, indeed, we
want not just our biological life but the purpose of our being
alive taken to the highest possibility of our functioning.

Beyond sleeping, dreaming and waking is a state in
which the 'I' is experienced to be 'empty' or utterly 'non-
material', never having been born and never capable of
dying—therefore, eternal. When this state is first clearly
experienced and accepted, a person can be said to be

---

awakened. An awakened person has something deep within, whether or not expressed in activity, which stands as a quiet reservoir for deep living.

If the 'awakened' state significantly penetrates past egoic limitations and is integrated at that level, it is called *realization.* Someone who is realized lives a life centered around that realization, even though that realization is not yet fully integrated into a continuous state. Nevertheless, a realized soul is noticeably empowered and his or her ability to gain from every situation in life usually stands out.

If 'realization' becomes permanent, it can be termed *liberation* (*moksha*, in Sanskrit). Despite how we may perceive someone in this state, also called 'cosmic consciousness,' a liberated soul is all the time self-aware and beyond the limited nature of the personality. Here, the nature of the "I" has been extended and deepened to infinity. In this blessed state, there is no inspiration to act, no doing and no control of any outcome, for the One Doer is inspiring and operating through such a soul. Such a one may seem very powerful, especially if the experience of 'liberation' is fairly new. A more integrated state of 'liberation' may seem far less impressive, though there is an ocean of divine potentiality constantly surrounding such a person.

Yet the duality of experience is not bridged until *enlightenment,* in which the infinity of the Self is perceived in everything, such that separation is solved in the union of Truth and Love in the open heart and clear mind. Such a soul perceives through at least one of the five senses every other soul and everything to be the one Reality, the sole Self, the vessel of infinity. That soul is a capable *guru.*

Is there more? While there are degrees of depth

to each of these seven states, such that we can say that the journey to Fullness never comes to an end, the other dimension of spiritual growth is described by the penetration of the *kundalini shakti*. The *shakti* is a motion independent of consciousness. One can be 'enlightened' and not have been fully penetrated by the primal ground force of Creation, whose purpose is to put through the nervous system the very impulse and power of Creation, which cleans the aspirant in favor of the most dynamic service. If states of consciousness demonstrate the essence of Life, the full-circle completion of the *kundalini shakti* demonstrates the expressive potential of Life. It is that which makes possible a *true human being*. One can be 'a true human being' without being 'enlightened' and visa versa. But why not have both!

Knowing what is possible prevents us from getting off the train of human development any sooner than we would elect. In this way we are empowered to achieve all that our heart can yearn for, and to be encouraged to continue on whatever quest is within us.

The Issue of Faith

Long journeys require great preparation.
The saga of how I came to be on this vessel would bore you.
I stand in the certainty of this ship landing in its port.
Already have I stood on terra firma
and am that steadfastness.

—Vishnu Datta—

Regardless of the spiritual path we choose, or the spiritual tool we use—even if it is the Divine gift of *Hari Om Tatsat Jai Guru Datta*—we will get only so far without faith. Faith is the strength necessary to continue our practice with clarity and sincerity in the face of obstacles and opposition. Bapu encourages us to have faith in God and/or *Guru*, faith in our practice and faith in ourselves.

Such faith grows with our experience. If we feel we are at all lacking in faith, the continued use of the *Hari Om Tatsat Jai Guru Datta mahamantra* will deliver the experiences required to organically build the faith we require.

Greater than belief is faith. According to a treasured ditty, "Belief clings; faith lets go. The former is taking as true something we read or hear, such as a verse of scripture. Faith, however, is based on what we have already experienced. When we experience something important—a certain kindness in a friend, for example—we can have at least some faith in his or her kindness. To have faith, we need to have been penetrated by an experience. Thus, belief is a relationship with a desirable state of affairs outside ourselves, while in faith that relationship has an internal basis.

Thus, we need experiences, and the Spontaneous

Meditation following the chanting of *Hari Om Tatsat Jai Guru Datta* is designed to bring us all the experiences we require. Through such experiences our faith is built, its foundation deepened and its castle with all its turrets fortified, heightened, and made more and more architecturally beautiful.

The Issue of Guidance

The One I love is not apparent
Yet I am that One's child.
I know so little, and that
Little is lessening into the night sky of my Beloved's gaze.

—Vishnu Datta—

We are, given the numerous—likely innumerable—layers of life, naïve or proudly stubborn if we feel we can get to our deepest heart's desire without guidance.

The pinnacle of human guidance is given the name 'Guru.' A true *guru* is an enlightened soul capable of imparting the light of knowledge and love to dispel the darkness of ignorance and fear. Such a soul, having the center of happiness and needing nothing for him- or herself, lives genuinely for the service of others. The infinity that is the revealed nature of a *guru* constantly informs his or her relationship with whomever has been drawn to this unique expression of divinity infused into humanity.

Bapu has said that everyone needs a *guru*. Those who have for numerous lifetimes dedicated themselves to *sadhana* may be advanced enough to have an ethereal *guru*, a great soul who is not incarnated in a human form. But most of us require a *guru* in a human body. To meet such a soul is a great fortune. The qualifications necessary for a true *guru* are that a) we know this soul knows us totally, b) we have experientially come to certainty that this soul has only our highest interest in mind and heart, c) we have faith that such a one is established in the highest state of human potential and d) we have no doubts that this person can capably guide us to that state.

Yet the very notion of 'guru' is mired in the media and in popular opinion due to the actions of some guides who, despite their responsibility for souls, evidently lack the spiritual integration necessary for constant non-manipulative service. Naturally, we may hold suspicions regarding this most-important relationship. To meet a Bapu, while rare, is to meet someone who dispels all such notions of limitation.

The universal *guru* is Reality itself, is Pure Consciousness, is the eternal Self and is not any body we can behold. Indeed, the true *guru* leads us to our own inner *guru*, which is the Truth in us constantly in communication.

Bapu, the most capable of *gurus*, does not offer himself as such, but suggests that, if we need a *guru*, that we take Sadguru, the Guru of Gurus, the very Lord as our very own *guru*. In this way, we will have the greatest of guidance, and Bapu's grace will be an automatic additional blessing.

Integrated Spiritual Progress

When the silent depths become bright
And the roiling surfaces darken into mystery,
I will know that everything is made of clear water
And will drown and declare myself the sea.

—Vishnu Datta—

The quality of integration is the measure of real maturity. This mantra brings that very blessing into the greatest of all arts—the art of living, which is the expression of our spiritual progress. Spiritual progress comes profoundly...yet slowly. "Slowly, slowly," says Bapu with a compassionate smile. It must be that way, so that the multitude levels of being all move in synchrony together. If one or more inner arenas purify and progress significantly beyond the others, then we can become imbalanced, which can bring us suffering or even feel dangerous.

Real progress is beyond fantasy, beyond guilt and beyond belief. In such a context of honesty and practicality, wisdom encourages us to understand that authentic progress is not the elimination of a difficulty, say 'fear', but the increase of the time between episodes, the lessening of their duration, and the decrease of the depth of disabling effects.

To value integration constitutes a vital dimension of wisdom.

PART IV

SADANA:
PRACTICE and
PRACTICALITIES

No one knows what sadhana is.

— Bapu —

Introduction

The more we know and experience that which fulfills us, the more we want to go deeper, to keep in mind and heart the reality we cherish. This motion towards the veracity of our true nature and our authentic service is called *sadhana* (spiritual practice). In order to reveal that which is true in all times and places, we keep turning our attention to what is deepest and most important within us. And, in so doing, we get this motion of spirit into our mind, into our emotional dimension and into our physiology.

Sadhana is our investment in the treasure we most want. Whatever the desired return—whether it be fame or prosperity or self-realization—investment is required of some time and some energy. Discipline is what makes a disciple. Thus, daily practice is the way of gaining maximum benefits.

Without doubt, the way of *Hari Om Tatsat Jai Guru Datta* is exceedingly simple, effortless and free of rules. Still some practical pointers will be wise to heed.

I. Daily Meditation

The simpler the way,

the more direct the connection.

Whatever doing might be instructed

Must fall away to allow for mastery.

—*Vishnu Datta*—

The state of meditation, which blessedly comes automatically after chanting this mantra, is the principal and most obvious gift of the *Hari Om Tatsat Jai Guru Datta* mantra. Since it comes without any doing, it is called Spontaneous Meditation—that meditation which comes naturally, spontaneously and without technique. This mantra—filled with energy and power, light and spirit, and wisdom and intelligence—works on anything and everything, such that all we need moves through it. *Hari Om Tatsat Jai Guru Datta* is an infinitely fluid intelligence which moves with each person in the same way that the Divine moves with humanity as a whole. Thus, this *mahamantra* represents the central intelligence that is working through humankind. The moment we try to add to its utter simplicity, we get significantly less, rather than more, of its benefits, since whatever we might add represents limitation, superstition, delusion and/or fear. *Hari Om Tatsat Jai Guru Datta* is complete, the universal gift.

To chant this mantra, one can simply clap and sing, *"Hari Om Tatsat Jai Guru Datta,"* repetitively in whatever melody for 5-10 minutes, then sit with eyes closed, and without touching anyone else. The usual time of daily meditation is 20-30 minutes, though one can meditate as long as desired—and twice a day, morning and evening, is a solid recommendation, given our daily routine and our need for energy when we go about our day and when we return home. While meditations of an hour or more are not uncommon for those drawn to this mantra, doing what time permits brings corresponding results.

Using a CD or cassette tape (of Bapu or anyone else chanting *Hari Om Tatsat Jai Guru Datta*) and singing in response is a popular way to chant the manta, then sitting in meditation. Or one can imitate the tape and sing by oneself or with a group.

Chanting and meditating in a group is often found to increase the power of the meditation and the experiences which can happen. The energy of the individuals in a group adds up sychronistically, thereby greatly enhancing the chant and meditation. Bapu does encourage us to chant vigorously, "like a child longing for its mother," he once said. Yet, if you are drawn into meditation even before the chanting is over, that motion is excellent and not to be avoided or prevented.

We can sit comfortably when we sit in meditation. Loosening whatever might be tight around the waist allows the subtle energies enlivened by this mantra to move more freely. Sitting up is recommended, since lying down is a physical signal for sleep. But we do not need to sit rigidly or overly erect. Sitting without back support does allow the subtle energies in the spine to move more freely, but if we require a backrest, then it is fine. Sadguru will take care of everything. There is no precise posture for sitting, for holding the hands or for any type of breathing. If you have a posture you prefer, by all means employ it. Meditating with animals remains a personal choice, though often (and unpredictably) they are drawn to the energy of this mantra and can compromise our stillness.

Again, there are no rules with this mantra, for *Hari Om Tatsat Jai Guru Datta* enlists neither dogma nor contexts of fear. The only detail that approaches a 'rule' is not to touch anyone else during the time of meditation, since to do so disturbs the 'energy envelope' surrounding a person in meditation. If you wish, you can begin with a prayer or speaking inwardly your intention. There is no need for incense or candles or photos, unless, of course, you wish to employ them.

After the chanting stops, simply be like a little child, go deep and enjoy. Do please remember to come out of meditation easily and gently, not opening the eyes too soon, and avoiding the urge to jump up quickly into activity. If meditation goes over whatever time limit has been established, this is always allowable.

Please also know that, life being full, meditation does not occur just with eyes closed. Bapu has said, "Meditation is not just like this" (imitating a meditative posture). Whenever we are contemplating the nature of life, of God, of our own reality, according to Bapu, we are engaged in meditation. Such an understanding of meditation helps us comprehend the outward and inward aspects of meditation as developing both our inner being and its manifest expressions.

II. Use of the *Hari Om Tatsat Jai Guru Datta* Mantra with Other Practices

Lord, I am not fickle, nor insincere.
You have given me more than one love, and
Since they are from You, I know
That all my lovers can love each other.

—*Vishnu Datta*—

It is a wise gift to authentically ask ourselves if whatever practice we are doing is actually working and if we have certainty that such a practice will develop us in all the ways we desire. If we do already employ and trust one or more spiritual practices, then we are fortunate. Even so, given the power and universality of this gift, this mantra should still be of significant benefit to us. Indeed, this *mahamantra* can be used in a way which empowers any practice we might faithfully employ.

The way to accomplish this benefit is to simply chant this mantra for 5-10 minutes before and after any practice we already sincerely enjoy. The blessings of *Hari Om Tatsat Jai Guru Datta* will grace the main practice, whatever it might be, of any practitioner.

III. Retreat

I had to quietly leave my known loves
To encounter love. I had to
Discretely disappear from my work to find my service.
In my silence, I found all musics joyfully arising.

—Vishnu Datta—

"You can't understand this mantra in only one experience," says Bapu. "Three days minimum," he advises. Thus, weekend and week-long retreats are being offered around the United States and Europe, as well as in India. On weekend retreats, for example, we would have at least five experiences of Spontaneous Meditation.

To come to *sahaj dhyan* and practice *sahaj dhyan yoga* on retreat significantly deepens our experience, not only due to the extra meditations, but also by virtue of the intention and the sychronistic effects of the group. The depth of experience on retreat is usually of a different order, representing a significantly deeper motion in us.

Daily meditation sets up a vital rhythm in our life. Regularity in this *sadhana* can hardly be overemphasized, if we indeed want to grow in the values of love, wisdom and peace. Periodic retreats add another longer and deeper wave of divine input, such that we then have yet another motion of rich support.

If there is not a retreat near you, retreats can happen anywhere significant interest in Spontaneous Meditation bubbles up.

IV. Use of the *Hari Om Tatsat Jai Guru Datta* Mantra in Daily Life:

Enough! I don't want you, Lord,
Only when the light comes or in the mists of evening,
Or only in weekend worship, or only in dream.
Be constant, Beloved, even in my sleep.

—*Vishnu Datta*—

During the day, this mantra may come to mind. We should consider it a gift. If we find ourselves repeating this mantra, excellent. If we wish or choose to do so, then, by all means, we are invited to engage in this movement of spirit. To repeat this mantra in a stressful or dangerous situation is to enlist the power of its blessings which stems from the Source of all blessings.

To find the mantra being repeated inside without our doing—on its own, as it were—is a very favorable development.

V. *Mala Jaapa*

As the moon is pulled round the seven-seas
Of the Earth, who is pulled round the pole of the Sun,
Who is pulled round the milk of the universe.
So am I pulling myself round my love for You.

—Vishnu Datta—

Life is whole, is holographic—not just 'inner' and
not merely 'outer.' Yet our longing for completeness is not a
confineable commodity, such that we wish for fullness only
on Tuesday nights or on the weekends or the summers. No,
our urge for totality is concomitant with our very humanity,
and the wholeness that lies as the deepest desire of our hearts
is infinitely beyond the sporadic and the part-time.

If our yearning for growth is tangible, then *mala
jaapa* practice is a definite aid. If our yearning is tangible
and acute, then we could say it is a must. *Jaapa* means
"remembering the name of the Lord." A *mala* is a rosary of
108 beads. The beads can be of any type, though *rudraksha*
(literally, "the tears of Shiva", which are seeds that grow
almost exclusively in the Himalayas) or tulsi seeds are the
most preferred.

The use of the *mala* is simple in concept: to say *Hari
Om Tatsat Jai Guru Datta* with every bead. One can say it
audibly (*manasika jaapa*) or inwardly (*vachika jaapa*), the
latter being the more potent. Going around once and saying
the mantra with each bead as you pull it to you constitutes
'one *mala*.'

The traditional way of holding the *mala* is to allow
it to hang in the crevice formed by the tip of the thumb

---

touching the tip of the ring finger of your right hand and then pulling the bead toward you with the tip of the middle finger. (This is called 'the deer mudra', for it looks like the face of a deer, with the pointer finger and the little finger forming respectively the left and right antlers.)

The *mala* is used with a *mala* bag, which is L-shaped, so that the bulk of the *mala* drapes down into the bag, thereby allowing the *mala* to be continually moved and allowing the energies of this practice to be contained in the *mala* bag.

The purpose of *mala jaapa* practice is to generate the subtle energies of the body, known as *kundalini shakti*. As per Bapu's very practical description, the action of the middle finger pulling each bead to reach the next bead generates a bit of friction, which is heat, which is light. This light is contained in the *gaumulke* and it is by grace transferred into the base of the spine, the seat of the latent "serpent power" of the *kundalini shakti* waiting to be awakened. The *shakti* power wants to rise through the subtle nexus points of nerve packages (*chakras*)in our body in order to purify our individual human nature so that the Divine can universalize us.

Moreover, Bapu has described the importance of *mala jaapa* as being that agent through which the 'residues of desire' are 'scrubbed away.' The act of looking outside ourselves for happiness and fulfillment, outside our own limitless nature, is a motion of veiling our true stature and beingness. These veils, residues and accumulations of built-up misdirected energy (ignorance) need to be removed if we are to function in the freedom and pristine qualities of our natural state. Yet, these veilings are sticky, viscous, and not unlike sludge built-up in a gas line or the hardening of arteries, such that some dynamically abrasive spiritual cleansing is required. *Mala jaapa* provides precisely this scrubbing action.

Please note: Doing *mala jaapa* for five to ten minutes is an authentic way into *sahaj dhyan* (Spontaneous Meditation), which is to say that we can enjoy Spontaneous Meditation by chanting the Hari *Om Tatsat Jai Guru Datta mahamantra* out loud in a group or by ourselves, or offer it out loud or silently on a *mala*.

Also, the main purpose of the *malas* is to lead to Spontaneous Meditation. Thus, if we ever find the *mala* has slipped from our hand, it is best then to simply sit in meditation, the dropping of the *mala* indicating that we are ready and that meditation wants to begin.

The instructions for *mala jaapa* are simple: to say as fast as possible, yet with clear pronunciation, the mantra with each bead. If doing more than one *mala*, when arriving at the end of the *mala* we do not cross the larger bead, called the 'Guru bead,' which represents infinity (and who can cross infinity!), but rather we then switch directions and move back the way we came.

The depth of this practice depends on the intensity with which we offer our *mala jaapa*.

Sankalp

On this seat in this place at this time,
I choose to give everything to you.
And so I remember the name of the One
Who has lead me to this love.

—*Vishnu Datta*—

There are two practices involving a *mala* and a *mala* bag which bear discussion, the first being the *sankalp*, which means 'determination" or 'vow'.

If we wish to do a *mala* practice for a specific purpose, whether for ourselves (say, for the optimum birth of our child) or for someone else (say, the healing of an illness), we can offer a *sankalp*. To make a *sankalp* means to offer a certain number of *mala*s for the same number of days for a given purpose that we clearly state each day before offering the *malas* for that day. This commitment requires our determination and constitutes a vow, which is *sankalp*. Thus, we could do three *malas* for three days or nine *malas* for nine days or thirteen *malas* for thirteen days, for example. Bapu has said that, if a loved one has passed on, we can offer twenty-one *malas* for twenty-one days (a practice especially important in the case of a suicide). Such a practice is not used as an entry into Spontaneous Meditation, since its benefits have been offered to some specific purpose for our own benefit or for another's.

To use the *mala* bag, which is L-shaped, is to hold the *mala* with one hand and allow its length to dangle into the bag itself. The bag is called a *gaumulke* (literally, 'the mouth of the cow,' the cow being considered as a blessing to the people of India) to indicate that this *mala* bag is filled with blessings. This practice allows the energy of our *mala jaapa* to build up in the bag and to benefit whoever is the recipient of the blessings of this *sankalp*.

Anusthan

Nothing works. Nothing is enough.
And yet I cannot stop longing to be nearer.
Take these recollections of the hint of closeness
And use them to enact this nothing that overtakes distance.

—*Vishnu Datta*—

The second arena of *mala jaapa* is called an *anusthan*. This practice is considered the fullest of *sankalps* and the strongest *mala* practice using the *Hari Om Tatsat Jai Guru Datta* mantra.

An *anusthan* is the daily offering of 52 *malas* (going around the 108-bead *mala* fifty-two times) for 52 days. Such a practice takes 1 ½ to 2 ½ hours a day, plus the *sahaj dhyan* afterwards,. As we get used to offering the *malas*, the smoothness of the practice goes faster and feels more and more natural.

Bapu has said that the reason for 52 *malas* is that there are 52 types of *kundalini shakti,* and that, therefore, they each get stimulated every day for this 52-day practice.

Therefore, the fullness of wisdom and physiological blessing is enlivened through this *anusthan* practice. Bapu has said that experience suggests that offering an *anusthan* "helps in making the mind…clean and pure and puts one on the path of spirituality." To offer a second or third *anusthan* "helps in stabilizing the mind and leads to the path of meditation."

This *jaapa* can be carried out anywhere. If we have a definite place where we can offer our *anusthan*, that place will feel empowered, electrified and pure.

The way of *mala jaapa* in an *anusthan* represents another step in familiarity with this mantra, in personal purification, and in depth of intimacy with the manifold mansions and terrains of our expanding inner nature.

PART V

QUESTIONS

To have questions is good.
Better is to have no questions.

— Bapu —

Introduction

The desire to understand is—as far as understanding can go—an authentic motion in the human spirit. The questions we do have deserve intelligent responses.

Bapu encourages us "to ask in meditation," which means to take our important queries into meditation and let Infinite Consciousness work through us in response, such that we have our own experience—by far the best 'answer' to whatever questionings we may offer.

There is a state of attainment in which all questions fall away and we have no more questions. Until then, may intelligent inquiries receive intelligent responses.

What does this mantra mean?

A mantra is utterly brimming with meaning and is as condensed an event as a 'black hole' in outer space. Even though a mantra does not 'mean' something—rather, it is something, meaning that it is that which it says, this intelligent question deserves a cogent response, for the intellect legitimately wishes to understand and comprehend.

Therefore, while a mantra represents a dimension that is beyond comprehension, let us approach the 'meaning' of the *Hari Om Tatsat Jai Guru Datta mahamantra* as follows:

Hari holds the Divine qualities of Love, Beauty and Bounty, and is represented in the Flower, and refers to all the Love and Consciousness that has ever taken a form. Jesus, Buddha, Krishna, Bapu—these are prime examples of *Hari*.

Om   holds the Divine qualities of Omniscience and Continuity throughout the ages, and is represented in the Conch, the Original Sound of the universe, and refers to the beginning, the middle and the finale of all Creation.

Tatsat   holds the Divine qualities of Reality and Pure Consciousness, and is represented in the Trident, and refers to the constant and omnipresent Reality of Truth that never changes.

Jai   holds the Divine qualities of Glory, Victory and Power, and is represented by the Discus, and refers to the all-victorious nature of the Supreme, Who is due every degree of glory.

Guru   holds the Divine qualities of Knowledge and Wisdom, and is represented in the Mace, the symbol of Divine authority, and refers to the Divine ability to transmute and transform the darkness of ignorance into the light of Knowledge.

Datta   holds the Divine qualities of Lover, Bestower and Blessing, and is represented in the *Mala,* and refers to the very nature of the Lord of Lords—to want to give everything the Lord is to everyone who longs for the fullness of Life.

Can anything fearful happen in meditation?

By virtue of the protection and integration of this *mahamantra*, nothing that we should fear can happen during meditation. However, this is not to say that we may not experience fear. Such an experience can occur after a particularly deep dive into our own nature, such that we may notice that we are barely breathing (because the body is so at rest that it requires only a minimum of breath). Our response may be that we suddenly feel we need more air, which we may then interpret as fear. In this example, any fear we might experience, while unnecessary, constitutes a purification of that fear.

At times in meditation I feel a definite heaviness in the head. Why?

The strong and subtle power of Sadguru begins even during the *dhun* to work inside the body and then continue even more deeply during Spontaneous Meditation. Heaviness in the head, body aches, feeling cool or even feverish (even though the body temperature remains normal) are all symptoms of the activity of this mantra as it enlivens the energy in the spine, from the perineum to the head, thereby revitalizing all aspects of our life.

During one meditation, I almost jumped off my seat. What happened?

The body, when a lot of subtle energy is moving rapidly, can move in order for that flow to be expressed. Such a motion is called a *kriya*. Whether our big toe experiences a pain, or we feel we are warm or cool, or one arm twitches noticeably--our physiology is trying to open so that the energy of the *shakti* can move and be free. This energy is, without doubt, completely intelligent, and whatever the manner it is arising is best treated with a welcoming, non-resistant attitude.

So much wants to happen in Spontaneous

Meditation—on so many levels. It is, therefore, wise to resist nothing in *sahaj dhyan* and to allow all that we are experiencing to move in just the way it is coming into expression from within.

What if I fall asleep in meditation?

Count sleep in meditation as a blessing. In every meditation, that which most needs to happen—given the state of our physiology—is happening. Thus, sleep is a gift, and sleep in meditation gives us a far deeper quality and degree of rest than sleep during a nap or during the night.

Of sleep in meditation, Bapu has said, "Major surgery requires general anesthetic." Far more is being accomplished in such sleep than we realize or likely can understand.

In meditation, I saw my parents in a car accident. I was so concerned! Will it really happen?

It is important to understand such an experience as the mercy of the Lord. Such an incident needed to happen but, through your meditation, it happened only on the level of your vision. Therefore, such an unfortunate event does not have to happen in the physical realm. This is a hint of Sadguru's love and mercy, that a physical accident was avoided by your *sadhana* and the necessity of its occurrence needed to occur only on the level of vision.

What would constitute the most rapid growth with this mantra?

The aspirant who wishes the fastest and fullest progress on the spiritual path will want to be regular in *dhun*

(chanting of this mantra) and *sahaj dhyan* (the Spontaneous Meditation that follows after chanting *Hari Om Tatsat Jai Guru Datta*) will want to have a daily *mala* practice and to make one or more *anusthans* (52 malas a day for 52 days), and will, along with making a retreat now and again, want to practice faithfully, with confidence and intensity.

I don't have any visions or flashy eperiences, but only peace. Is that okay?

Most certainly. Bapu says that is what this mantra is most meant to give. Peace is wonderful, the nature of life, and you are fortunate.

Are you saying that this mantra is really better than all the other divine gifts that have come to human kind?

The critical time in which we live is bringing from the Divine many gifts. Our planet needs them all. The *Hari Om Tatsat Jai Guru Datta mahamantra* has not been bequeathed to humanity to assume a position of 'best' or even 'better'. Rather, this is a motion of what is 'appropriate'. We are moving into an era with new energies and possibilities. This mantra has been 'crafted' for exactly the times in which we live, and its blessings are unprecedented. It is for everyone, though not everyone will be drawn to this gift. Whosoever is drawn will be fortunate, without doubt.

Since this mantra is so protective, I will always feel safe, right?

This mantra is totally protective, yes. And you will always be safe. However, you may not always *feel* safe. We cannot expect to be led out of limitations and boundaries and always feel safe. This person we call 'myself' is not just this physical body. Since life is layered, we have other bodies—a mental or psychic body, an emotional body and other even subtler bodies. The emotional body needs to be purified, as does our physical body, so that we can be free in our feelings, to experience without fear all that life wants to show us. On the way to such freedom, expansiveness and fearlessness, we will pass through some senses of limitation, contraction and fear. And at some point we will part from this limited physical body. And at that moment, we will without doubt be guided and assisted by the Lord of Lords and all the *Siddhas* and great beings associated with this mantra. Therefore, whoever comes to this mantra with faith and sincerity will, despite whatever feelings arise, always be safe.

> *In the past, I've had a bad experience with*
> *spirituality from a false teacher. How can I*
> *come to faith and sincerity in this mantra?*

Because this is a deeply spiritual time on our planet, there are many gifted souls who are fully capable and sincere who can be of deep and direct service to us. However, there are also many gifted souls who are either not capable, or not as capable as they say they are, and/or who are insincere and even so misguided as to be dangerous. The wounds due to such involvement can be very subtle and take years to heal.

This mantra is straight from God to you. It is so deeply and fully protective. And its ability to heal is unfathomable—one can know how deep only after opening to one's God-given depth as a person. Yet, understandably you are reluctant to take anyone's word about these important

---

parameters. Your having asked the question suggests some willingness, despite your difficult past experience, to move forward, to honor your soul in its yearning for something true, non-manipulative, uncomplicated and authentic. Therefore, try just listening to this mantra. Its effects are significant enough that just listening, without trying to sing along, to the *dhun* (chant) of *Hari Om Tatsat Jai Guru Data* are very gifting. Then, if you are moved to do so, at some point chant along. And, whenever the time feels right, close your eyes and enjoy Spontaneous Meditation. You can begin with just a minute or two. Maybe then five minutes, then ten minutes. Go at your own pace, and follow your inner sense of direction.

What about the judgments of my family and friends?

When we embark in a direction (inner or outer) that holds great promise and potential, others—often especially those close to us—may question our choice and motivation...both in legitimate concern for us and all too often in defensiveness of their own viewpoint. Our relationship with ourselves, and with God, is subtler, more powerful, more primal, more intimate and more consequential than our relationship with anyone else, even our parents or spouse or children. We owe this most important relationship all that we can offer—in the face of criticism or even outright antagonism. We need never be resentful in the face of the concerns of those close to us. Yet, we do have a choice of whether to move in our inspiration or in the inspiration of others.

Is this gift for children?

In the 1980s, Bapu would offer *Hari Om Tatsat Jai Guru Datta* in local schools. The students would chant the mantra and go into meditation and, whenever a suspicious administrator would end the meditation, the youths would come out crying, "Why did you bring us out of that peace?" and they would plead to return into that state.

Yes, this gift is for youths as well as adults. If a child can understand the need for peace, then this *sahaj dhyan* can be a great grace in his or her life. Moreover, children appreciate their parents practicing this meditation and growing in its benefits, since the experience of meditation serves to make the parents more loving and peaceful.

A young friend when she was age ten went with her father to Girnar Sadhana Ashram and met Bapu. She, raised as a devout Catholic, was reading a 'comic book' about one of the great epics of India—the story of Lord Ram and his wife Sita and their extraordinary ally Hanuman, king of the monkeys who is the epitome of service and devotion. During her time at the ashram, in meditation she saw Hanuman pulling his chest apart to reveal his heart, which contained the faces of Ram and Sita. She found herself weeping in meditation, overwhelmed with such selfless beauty, especially because it reminded her so concretely of the sacred heart of Jesus. Perhaps we can conclude that *sahaj dhyan* brings out the best in us, and, because children are so innocent, that they can especially be nurtured and their essence be revealed by this meditation.

Is it true that I don't have to give anything up to enjoy this mantra?

This *mahamantra* works in the same way as the Divine—supporting each of us exactly where we are and moving us in ourselves on our journey to fullness. Therefore, there are no requirements to begin and enjoy the blessings of this Divine gift other than to use it.

If we utilize this mantra, we will be benefited. Those benefits will deepen us, will focus as well as expand us, and will mature us. As we grow, our beliefs, our behavioral habits, and our energies will also likely deepen, congeal, expand and mature.

I am neither smart nor well-read, and yet still have deep longings for God. Can someone like me still gain enlightenment.

Book knowledge or any kind of outer information will not fulfill us, and thus it is not a requirement for fulfillment. This *mahamantra* is not based on human scales of intelligence, but on the fact that you are a soul. All that you need to know will come to you through its regular and confident use. Indeed, you may receive deep intelligence in meditation that will astound the world. All intelligence comes from the Source of Intelligence, Who gave this mantra to Bapu.

If I'm ill, can I still use this mantra?

Most certainly, for this mantra gives us exactly what we currently need, including the healing rest that meditation is designed for. The experience may be one of falling into sleep...again and again, which is precisely what we require

---

when we are dealing with illness. Sleep in meditation is in an entirely different category of rest—in degree and quality—than regular sleep during the night and, therefore, is not meant to replace a good night's sleep. Yet the kind of rest gained from 'sleep in meditation' is incomparable and enormously beneficial to any state of illness.

Similarly, pregnancy will be wonderfully served with this mantra, as well.

The future looks fearful…What do I do?

We cannot do anything about the future. We can act only in the present. Yet, no matter what is to come, this mantra will pour its blessings into anyone who utilizes it faithfully. The protection, the guidance, the integration and the strength that come with this mantra will—along with the Lord of Lords, Bapu and all the Siddhas—be as solid an insurance policy as is possible. Bapu has said that the Supreme never lets go of anyone who comes to this mantra.

Who is Bapu?

He is Shri Punitachariji Maharaj, the most integrated of human beings and someone who has incorporated true human beingness into the highest state of consciousness and a lifetime of service. He was the highest order of renunciate until 1981. At that time Sadguru requested that he marry. Now he is in the *rishi* tradition, a family man. His consort, Guru Ma Shri Shalaja Devi (Mataji) is, according to Bapu, *Yogamaya*—the power of manifestation itself throughout creation. Together they have raised a son Lalaji and a daughter Ummaji. Bapu stands for the fullness of dedication to Absolute Reality and the completeness of human existence. The founder of Girnar Sadhana Ashram said, "For me, I do not like this kind of place" (motioning to the ashram buildings); "I like this kind of place" (pointing to the hearts of those sitting before him). Such is his true habitat.

Bapu is a Datta *avatar* (an incarnation of Lord Dattatreya), a *siddha parusha* (a perfected servant) and a master of *sadhana*. Though the most capable of *gurus*, he does not offer himself as a *guru*, saying for those who wish a *guru* to take Sadguru Datta, the Guru of gurus, as the *guru*. Yet he is a true guide to Self-Realization, the highest development possible, when one is no longer limited by the body. "I am just an operator," Bapu has said: "If you want Jesus, if you want Ram or Krishna, if you want Buddha, if you want Allah…" and then he makes a motion like a telephone operator to indicate that he will plug us in to whatever we want.

To understand Bapu is to see someone who is entirely empty, simple and more childlike than an infant. He is everywhere and 24 hours a day is attending to the needs of others throughout the universe. "I am not this form," says Bapu, "and this is my science." Even his age is mysterious, and he has said, "If I said how old I am, no one would believe me."

He asks for nothing from us except our *sadhana*, and the only payment he will accept is our giving up our pain, our doubts and worries. Once, traveling with friends, rather that taking the middle back seat as was his habit, he took a side position. That trip resulted in Bapu's car being hit by another driver just where Bapu was sitting, fracturing the sage's arm. In 'taking the hit' for someone else, he demonstrates his friendship, courage and care.

This is his last life, and, before merging into Sadguru, he is repaying even the smallest of kindnesses ever done to him.

Is it possible to meet Bapu?

Yes, it is quite possible to meet Bapu. Despite his greatness, he is present to whoever comes to Girnar Sadhana Ashram, most especially if they come for the purpose of *sadhana*. He is not unavailable. Of him, a friend has noted, "Of the learned he is the most learned, and of the common he is the most common." If you are interested in visiting, it would be wise to email the ashram with the dates of your visit, to make sure that Bapu is not away with family or offering this mantra. It is noteworthy that he is, these days, spending more time in his cave (below his house at the ashram), doing a "big work" for the world. Yet he usually comes out at least on Sunday afternoons for *darshan*.

It is also quite possible to meet him inside, in meditation. If you wish, you can ask in meditation for such a meeting. Because Bapu is not his form, you might want to specify the kind of meeting that interests you. As always, expectations hinder, rather than promote, optimum results.

How long will fulfillment take?

This unanswerable question depends on many factors: sincerity, faith, character and destiny, as well *sadhana*. However 'long' it takes, it is worth all our dedication, for our only other choice is to continue suffering. We do live in extraordinary times, an era in which we can, if we wish, make tremendous strides in spiritual growth—such that we should think that the ultimate goal of all human existence can be ours in this very lifetime.

Do I have to believe in God to benefit from this mantra?

The existence of God may be long and well debated, but this is only because the Supreme is the summation of everything that exists infused with the infinite Source. Thus, God, known by so many names, exists beyond all names and has no preference for what name we might prefer. Indeed, God does not care if we believe in 'God'—only that we come to the fullness of Life. That fullness exists beyond all limitations. If believing there is no God arises from a limitation in us, we will eventually be moved beyond that boundary. If we have beliefs, positive as they might be, which limit God, we will eventually be moved beyond those boundaries. Belief in God is not required to come to or enjoy the blessings of *Hari Om Tatsat Jai Guru Datta*, despite that this *mahamantra* has come from the mouth of God.

Is what you are offering a religion?

The *Hari Om Tatsat Jai Guru Datta mahamantra* is pre-religious, its intention representing the centrality of Reality prior to the impulse of religion. *Hari Om Tatsat Jai Guru Datta* can impart all that religion is designed to bring, but it does so 'secretly', for its gift presupposes no inherent dogma or theology or philosophy—even though it is philosophically, theologically and spiritually profound. This mantra can be used independently of religious involvement, for it is known as 'the path of the yogi mystics', or it can be used in support of any of our great religious traditions. In many cases it has inspired an aspirant to embark on or go deeper into a given religious tradition.

Must I eventually believe in Reincarnation?

We are not our beliefs, whether they are limiting ones or de-limiting ones. Every belief represents a point of view, and every point of view represents, of necessity, some limitation. In the West, the notion of reincarnation is not generally held by the three 'religions of the book.' However, if reincarnation is 'true', then we might infer that at some point we will encounter that truth. Yet, even if we were to have an experience in meditation that seems to directly confirm the reality of reincarnation, it is still up to us what we wish to believe. Bapu may speak of past lives, but neither he nor Sadguru Datta is interested in convincing anyone of this insight. Life does all the teaching, each life is unique, we will be presented with all that we need to learn, and we will learn whatever we want.

What makes for real spiritual maturity?

Integration of all that is Divine and all that is human, of all that is Heaven and all that is Earth—beyond all dualities and pairs of opposites—in the constant service of all spiritual journeyers stands as the ideal of human potential and constitutes what might be termed 'complete spiritual maturity'.

PART VI

EXPERIENCES

Love is the only rational act of a lifetime.
All else is nonsense and falderol.

— Bapu —

Introduction

The great *Hari Om Tatsat Jai Guru Datta* mantra comes directly from the Source of Experience and leads, ultimately, beyond all experiences to that ultimate Source. Yet, on the way to the finale of human potential, experiences play a vital role whose importance is real. Experiences arising from and gifted by this mantra are intimate events, indeed, representing the intersection of the personal and the universal, such that no two persons experience the exact same experience, which are each more unique than snowflakes.

Experiences can guide us, console us, confirm a state that before was hazy or not well-integrated, challenge us, purify us, and inspire us.

What follows are experiences selected for their utility in describing, at least in part, some of the countless effects of this Divine gift.

"My first experience I warmed all over. As if being protected by something--and blessed. The heat or light lasted much longer than the meditation lasted. I can only describe it as intense healing directly from God. Very safe. Blanketed in love, care and compassion." G. C., Chicago, IL

Commentary: This individual's first experience with Hari Om Tatsat Jai Guru Datta exhibits the aspects of energy (heat/light), protection, blessing, healing and love of this mahamantra. It is not unusual that someone has a profound experience in their very first Spontaneous Meditation.

"In my first meditation with *Hari Om Tatsat Jai Guru Datta*, I felt a great deal of energy in my body, especially around my head, as if I were wearing a protective helmet. It felt heavy, yet good. Inside I felt peace. It was a strong experence."   H. L. Omaha, NE

Commentary: This person's experience is fairly common with this mahamantra, even during the very first meditation. The 'helmet' of energy is a hallmark of being connected to the Divine through this mantra. And the peace and energy in the body are also, even if it is someone's first-ever meditation, often reported.

"During my first experience with the mantra, we were all soothed by the experience and elated at its conclusion. We followed the tape carefully that night, and I remember most the pace increasing and a feeling of speed and intensity, but without chaos or fear—in a whirling gathering of energy exceeding that of the people in the room. I knew I was responding to the voices of the men and women on the tape, and that we were separated in time, and yet we were somehow floating together, all together in a place both present and separate - a place of clear vision and joy. Sitting quietly together, basking in the post chanting space, I felt strong hints of my place in a great universe. I carry the mantra with me. I feel protected by it, finding myself speaking it in my mind or softly in voice, when I'm fearful."   J. C., Madison, WI

Commentary: Here, in another first-time experience with this mantra, the individual experiences what every soul wishes to experience, yet one which can elude even veteran aspirants on the spiritual journey--something of the vast interconnectedness of all life, such that we feel we belong and are an important part of the great saga of Creation.

✻

"While I haven't practiced the meditation as much as I should, so I haven't had any great experiences, here is what happens when I do it. I have tried other meditation techniques but none of them ever made my mind quiet. Within five minutes I would be day-dreaming. I also would become restless just after ten minutes -- and ten minutes of meditation felt like I had sat for half an hour. But when doing the *Hari Om Tatsat Jai Guru Datta sahaj* meditation, my mind gets "thoughtless" and peaceful immediately and sitting for half an hour seems like only ten minutes."

P. P., South Chicago, IL

Commentary: Whatever we invest in this meditation, the returns—while commensurate with our investment—are remarkable, nonetheless. This experience is an excellent commentary on sahaj dhyan (Spontaneous Meditation) and the state of meditation it produces—without effort or method.

✻

"Dear Bapu, I have benefited extremely from your mantra *Hari Om Tatsat Jai Guru Datta*. There is a man in India…who has been doing black magic on me for the past 12 years. The attacks started in…1992, till last June 26, 2004.

I used to pray to God to…give me protection, and exactly one month ago I accidentally found your website of Lord Dattatreya. I have been using this mantra for exactly one month, and the attacks stopped. I have lots of energy in my body. I have been working for 20 days without a break and no signs of tiredness. Whenever I experience any obstacle, I take this mantra, and I overcome the obstacle…."

M.G., Panama City, Panama

Commentary: Here is a prime example of the protection that this great mantra affords, as well as the energy to enact our lives as we live them day by day. This individual is receiving significant benefits even from learning about Hari Om Tatsat Jai Guru Datta over the internet.

❋

"Chanting the mantra…has brought me much greater clarity and serenity, for which I am ever grateful. Additionally, I call on its soothing tones when I sense a potential for danger and trust that its blessing - its ability to channel me into a greater awareness of divinity - will see me through any challenge. …Last year (2003) I was traveling with a friend out…toward Mt. Delenbaugh …on dirt roads when weather conditions turned for the worst. …I calmly chanted the mantra with supreme confidence that we would never be faced with any serious danger…in spite of the fact that my friend was QUITE certain we were in for major problems of every sort. Indeed, we made it through the storm with no trouble…. Peace and serenity expand in my life when I am faithful with the chanting of this sacred mantra."

G. S. J. Hurricane, UT

Commentary: The peace available in this mantra is unlimited. Here again, the sense of protection in every situation is a striking benefit.

✳

"I sat down, not wishing for anything, so I asked God to bless me in any way he felt I needed. I had lost my son at age 22 a few years before. When the chanting of the mantra stopped, I had the vision of my son at every year. He was coming to me and smiling and hugging me with each vision. This experience was very powerful and brought such emotional release that it will be with me forever."

D. B., Crestone, CO

Commentary: The Lord of Lords knows exactly what we need. Such a healing cannot be found in any of the healing arts--except through Divine blessing. Again, this was this person's first experience of this mantra.

✳

"My most predominant experience with this mantra is love, the deep sense of a vast love that is for everyone, a feeling of connectedness and softness which often brings me to tears of beauty and awe. But once, I fell into meditation even before the chanting of the mantra. During this meditation, a lot of stuff came up. I had been praying for self-knowledge, to become more aware of my limitations. Inside, I saw more deeply than ever before my lack of love, where I'm afraid to love. I know this goes way back, certainly to my birth, which was horrific and lasted for days. So I could see a block to love in my personality and I wept throughout the *dhun* and meditation. Yet, afterwards, I felt washed with insight and gratitude."   N. S., Crestone, CO

Commentary: The process of purification, especially in souls as sincere as this aspirant, is experienced as a definite blessing. "Everything that has gone in must come out," says Bapu. And it is not uncommon in those familiar with this mahamantra to fall spontaneously into meditation during or even before the dhun (chant).

❈

[It is first important to mention that, prior to this experience, I had never been taught anything about yogic postures or yogic breathing.] "During one morning meditation…I found myself having a hard time getting enough air. I didn't feel suffocated, but simply wished my lungs had capacity for more air. I felt the urge to hold my breath for long periods of time. Even after holding the breath for several minutes, I found myself still needing more air…and the urge to force my back to round out in an effort to stretch the capacity of my lungs. Then, after breathing in, I pushed my chest forward to lock the breath in for some time. This process continued…and eventually I felt the urge to lean forward on my hands and knees with my back bending up and out with my head down on the inhale and then switching to my stomach down…. It felt so good. I felt I could hold my breath forever. …To stretch my body, I went from posture to posture on my hands, knees, feet, toes, back, bending and stretching every muscle in my body intricately. I remember one posture on the floor with my legs bent at the knees with my feet tucked under me, and I was able to lean all the way back with my head, shoulders and back flat on the floor. ...But there was no pain. It felt like relief. I was intuitively instructed with each different position to turn my hands, fingers, arms, legs or toes in such a specific manner so as to stretch or bend a specific muscle. I knew a healing was taking place. ...This process lasted several hours, for many months afterwards, and even now occasionally with continued practice of the mantra. ...I felt the urge to laugh out loud because I had never been able to stretch my body into such difficult positions. I later learned that each posture I had assumed had a name, and that the different breaths were called Pranayama and each had a specific purpose. ...I didn't need a class or a book to learn them. This mantra awoke not only the outer yoga but also the inner yoga in me. Sitting silently with the energy invoked by the vibrations of the mantra allowed my inner teacher to guide me to what is natural and vital within every human being. It catalyzed the spiritual and scientific dimension that was dormant for so long."

A. L., Glen Garden, NJ

Commentary: The power, the shakti, of this mantra is so integrating and full that it can—without disturbing the state of meditation—allow someone to move in ways the body could not duplicate outside of that sahaj dhyan, so that the energies being released get optimumly distributed throughout the nervous system. Spontaneous asanas (yogic postures) and pranayamas can happen in order to get the essential breath deeper into the body, for the breath brings fresh healing energy and enlivens the physiology as often nothing else can—very invigorating.

"Most of my spontaneous meditations following the *Hari Om* chanting are simply very deep, quiet, peaceful experiences, such that I feel refreshed and resolved afterward. I usually sleep well those nights. These are great gifts to one with as active a mind as myself. Profoundly simple gifts of grace." K. S., Crestone, CO

Commentary: Experiences through this mantra do not have to be extraordinary or flashy to be profound and transformative. We see with this Spontaneous Meditation that deep experience in meditation have important effects in activity...and, in this case, in sleep.

"In my first experience of '*Hari Om*', I enjoyed singing the mantra, and especially the drumming. I had no particular expectations; however, when all the chanting stopped, I heard a voice compelling me to reach up: "Stretch!" I was on my knees and lifted my hands above my head and reached. Again and again I was told to stretch! I kept stretching and reaching up, until all of a sudden I felt every vertebra in my neck down to my sacrum adjust! It was the greatest and best adjustment I have ever received. For two days afterwards, I walked between the thoughts. I was in bliss like never before." S. B., Crestone, CO

Commentary: Through the directness of this mahamantra, the Supreme works in ways that we can understand. In this manner, a clear and unique relationship

is built between the Divine and the aspirant. Sadguru interacted with personal intimacy in the way which would speak most deeply to this individual, who is a Doctor of Chiropractic.

�֍

"There was, on my first experience of this mantra, an experience of peace. Then came sadness, deep sadness. I would dip back into the peace, and then this deep sadness would return, and this back and forth of peace and sadness continued for most of the meditation." K. L., St. George, UT

Commentary: This simple experience is revealing of the mechanics of meditation, which are no different than the mechanics of life itself. The two pistons of the engine of personal progress—the urge toward peace and the urge toward purification (so that greater peace can be enjoyed and integrated—are clearly at work here. This person feels sadness, but only after experiencing peace, then dipping back again into peace which then is followed by more deep sadness. These two strokes of peace and purification are both necessary and both profound gifts of meditation.

✖

"I have seen visions. The most pronounced of the visions, at first, appeared as an octagon of pure light, which became a diamond of light that moved through a tunnel and then became a tiny dot of light, which disappeared into timelessness and spacelessness. I came out of meditation smiling, feeling quiet and at ease." M. G., St. Louis, MO

*Commentary: Visions are not uncommon experiences
with this mantra. They are not required for spiritual growth,
and yet can bring not only clarification and direction, but
also a closer and more intimate relationship with what
is lasting and real. Usually they are accompanied by the
blessing of an inner state of peace.*

❋

"On many occasions when I'm in the space of my
mind being silenced and still, I see a colored orb of purple/
blue with the same brilliance as a flame. The orb is right in
front of me. It pulsates slightly bigger and smaller. At some
point the inner part of the orb would turn gold. The gold
would pulse out larger to envelop the purple/blue, but then
the purple/blue would appear in the center. It would then
pulse out to the perimeter and the gold would appear in the
center. This cycling…would continue for some time. I often
interpret this purple/blue as a representation of my higher
self, and I also feel that the gold is some manifestation of
divinity. I feel that we are dancing together in the form of
these pulsing colors within the orb".   M. F., Crestone, CO

*Commentary: Visions, whether of persons or events
or insights into the inner workings of consciousness on planes
more subtle than our physical reality, can be deeply revealing
and constitute experiences that we can return to again
and again for meaning, inspiration and encouragement.
While they can seem 'film-like', whatever we might 'see' in
meditation usually also 'speaks' to us in very deep ways.*

❋

"After chanting *Hari Om Tatsat Jai Guru Datta* with a small group of people, we sat for meditation and I experienced a deep peace and tranquility. Then I had a vision of light emanating from a fluorescent light that I saw within me. I internally saw electrons traveling through the bulb and striking gas molecules, which resulted in the light. Then I sensed that beyond the energy of this light was a greater power—an unseen force that motivates and empowers the energy and movement of electrons striking gas in a tube. This force is much more powerful yet subtle than energy or movement as we typically experience it: It is pure intentionality and power that brings about phenomena that we can actually perceive. Now, often during my daily life, I am reminded of the power and intentionality that is behind and beyond my experience, which empowers such phenomena—including even my own breath and life."   T. P., Davis, CA

Commentary: The revelations of Infinite Intelligence can show us—whether we are primarily artistic or scientific—any and all the layers of life and their inner workings. Through the blessings of this mantra, we come to realize that to know about something 'out there' is to find out about our own inner workings, for we find not two separate universes, but different expressions of the same mechanics of manifestation. There are not two realities—an inner and an outer—but only one. To see the nature of light is also to see that we are the light.

※

"In 2000, during the meditation I had a vision. The vision was... "You must allow yourself to be devoured by the spider in order to become part of the Web of Life."

When I moved to Hurricane, Utah, I was all-consumed by Spider Woman and spiritual aspects of the spider. On, 8/9/02, I noticed that Lord Datta who is the prominent deity for Bapu has 6 arms & 2 legs. In other words, it is also a representation of Spider Woman! Since then, I have found many other spiritual connections around the world associated with the spider. We are all connected; we are all part of the web of life."   R. U. Hurricane, UT

Commentary: Here is another type of vision, that which brings inner information and stitches together meaning in such a way that our entire journey is deepened. The person who received this touchstone experience has, with this thread of new understanding, experienced a quantum leap in his work of discovering and deciphering petroglyphs.

✽

"This experience occurred when Bapu came to our house and had me sit in front of him for *dhun* and *dhyan*. It was the first time I had heard him say to chant this mantra like a child longing for its mother—and this created a different dynamic in me. We started the chanting and, as it built in speed, very simple images came to me. And I felt as though I was chanting the mantra not only for myself and my family and those close to me, but that a circle of connection began to expand in time and space. A succession of images came—of children in poverty, of people in prison. I was now chanting on behalf of the entire human family. And it went beyond humanity to the entire natural world. Each individual image stood as a wholeness—until the entire wholeness of life was present. Then, because my root tradition is Christianity—the final image was of Christ on the Cross. My own heartfelt desire transcended my individuality and embraced all of Creation. My experience was linked with that of Christ through this mantra."   T. H., Austin, TX

Commentary: In this powerful example of universal love, we can glimpse the all-embracing nature of this mantra which, because it is a direct gift from God, stands in solidarity with all souls in their need, with all of Creation.

"During the 1999 retreat in Crestone with Bapu, the group of well over one hundred souls was sitting in well-defined rows. I saw, though my eyes were closed, the Divine presence of protective energy move as a light up and down each of the rows, transforming our energetic bodies into bodies of light. I felt this to be happening without exception to each of us. The feeling was one of tremendous orderliness and a strength of grace that I could feel throughout my being."   I. S., Crestone, CO

Commentary: The blessings of this mantra are beyond measure. What actually occurs in any session of Spontaneous Meditation is neither perfunctory nor rational, but constitutes the direct blessing of the Lord in manifold ways, and its action and benefits are unfathomable. This individual happened to glimpse, with eyes deeper than our physical eyes, some hint of the motions of Divine grace.

"In 2001, I had a vision of Lord Dattatreya. Bapu laughed and said, "It took me forty years!" Recently, when doing the mantra, I become very aware of Dattatreya. Such a sense is so hard to describe, but there is a great feeling of love and compassion. And there is no fear—like everything is taken care of. The mind settles down because there is nothing to worry about. There is only joy and love. But I am aware of a being and some celestial place. It's like driving along and cresting a hill, and suddenly there is a vista in front of you. The mind might wander, but when I come back to my heart, I'm aware of this amazing vista. When actually chanting the mantra, there is a flow of energy that goes out and comes back—love and gratitude, which is very strong, moving to the Lord and being returned. Now, whenever I read of or hear about Sadguru Datta, I weep. The tears take me so deep into myself. They are tears of gratitude, joy, knowingness, being—they go beyond words."

B. W., Boulder, CO

Commentary: The Lord is so kind, so wondrous—and so actual. There is a state of attainment in which the sadhaka weeps whenever the Divine is mentioned. Such a state of affairs is most fortunate and can be given to communicate with an aspirant that the connection with the Supreme is not only vital and real but also undying.

※

"While meditating in the Solar Dome of the Sri Aurobindo Learning Center of Savitri House, a clear but urgent message came from the Mother, regarding the mantra. She said, "This mantra is an accelerated spiritual discipline, that in repeating it one clears the inner channels, unlocks mental and emotional barriers held within the chakras, and above all clears the physical and subtle physical bodies [etheric] in order for greater clarity to enter. This is done through the power of the truth of the Divine Structure of our nature, and anchoring it in our consciousness more and more firmly."

She urged me to work with and to help in the furthering of this mantra to the best of my capacities, and thus gave her blessings.

At another special evening *dhun* at the Desert House for my Aurovillian friends, during the chant and again during the meditation I saw Bapu, not physically present with us, from a distance shooting a sword of brilliant white light into the gathering. I saw how this sword of light chipped away and melted and cut all the blockages and resistances we have within ourselves. It worked on us intensely to make us much more receptive, malleable."   M. P., Montebenichi, Italy

Commentary: These experiences speak to what Bapu says to those who already have a guru—that they simply ask their guru to reveal what this mantra is, that if it is true to show its truth.

※

"I was visiting Girnar Sadhana Ashram and had a major personal decision to make. I asked Bapu about it and he said, "Tomorrow in meditation, I will help you." I hardly slept at all that night. During meditation the next morning, I went to a place which is familiar and very deep, a place I experience almost as the bottom of the ocean, so all-encompassing it is. I then experienced going beneath that known and magnificent place to a new, more open place where I was shown a perspective that the decision I had to make didn't matter. No choice I could make was more important than another, and there couldn't possibly be a mistake. The truth was that the real 'I' of me was in motion beneath whatever space that decision occupied. I saw that this decision would play out through cause and effect without touching this place I was viewing it all from. I drew, and still draw, enormous strength from this experience."

N. L., Snowmass, CO

Commentary: This mantra is coming from and returning us to a 'place' beyond the fear-creating pairs of opposites, a place of wisdom and mercy and fullness. The above experience hints at how everything is disappearing from its seemingly limited context and being re-experienced as unity, a 'place' of non-separation, which is the essence of love, strength and peace. Everything is disappearing into the Lord.

✻

"The first time I experienced the *Dhun* and meditation I felt myself in a state of nothingness, which was very clam and peaceful. Then suddenly after awhile of "nothingness" appeared a profound radiance of Light, which I somehow knew was the Being of Christ. I felt that I was receiving a blessing. After the meditation was over and people were sharing their experiences, I shared what happened to me. A few people shared with me that when they first experienced this mantra/meditation they too had felt and seen the image of

Christ. ...During the chanting phase of the *Dhun*/meditation I have experienced, sometimes, a deep breathing rhythm in my heart center, which feels balancing and comforting. Usually nowadays my experience is of deep peace with no visuals at all. I feel the depth of peace carried with me throughout the day benefits my ability to stay centered no matter how stressful life is."   A. F., Rockland, ME

Commentary: It is not unusual for people to experience something of the great guides of humanity. Indeed, even if we have a specific religious allegiance, we may encounter a representative of another spiritual tradition. Bapu explains that we have had many lifetimes prior to this one, and past relationships may show up during sahaj dhyan in this life. But more important is the sense of deep peace. "The visuals" may well fall away, but the peace is that which can uphold every experience, both in meditation and in our daily lives.

❋

"For many months my early *Dhun* experiences contained a lot of dancing; ...while chanting I would be sitting and perhaps swaying a bit side to side, but in my mind's eye I would be dancing. In my body sense I felt that I was dancing, sometimes dancing around the room. Many times I would feel as though I was dancing with one or more snakes. Even though I would only mildly rock or sway in my physical body, my energy body was dancing. I feel this helped move the energy in my...energy channels. The dancing felt old and familiar...and I always felt quite exhilarated afterwards."   M. F, Crestone, CO

Commentary: This experience hints at the great energy available through this mantra, an energy present within every person, but hidden—until it starts to be awakened. And through this mantra, the energy is awakened in an integrated manner. Such energy, while beyond the rational mind, is not chaotic, as this experience indicates, but rhythmic and meaningful.

"There are no words that can describe the truest value or essence or meaning of this mantra. The waves of insight and healing that come through it are so sublime, and altering. It's like a vehicle or a bridge that links me to the Source and the Fullness of All That Is. When people ask if I do this mantra practice, I almost laugh, because it's more like the mantra "doing" me. It might have looked like I decided to attend gatherings where I could learn/experience this way, and perhaps my choice to do that was somehow instrumental, but over time it became clear that I was reeled in like a fish on a line. I study and practice other paths, too, but "the mantra" (for lack of a better phrase to describe the whole matrix to which it relates) provides a kind of organizing system and a potency for all the pieces in the mix. Even through periods when I don't "use" or pay attention to the mantra –it still seems to be operating underneath and throughout. I am so grateful."

B. R., Crestone, CO

Commentary: This soul, who has been sincerely practicing for some time, sees into the wholeness of this mantra and its blessings, and understands that in this mantra there is no bias for one way or another way into the fullness of existence. Rather, this mantra blesses all efforts and all understandings.

�֎

"In one 5-hour meditation, I encountered a spiritual hopelessness that for 20 years I had carried, but had just ignored. Its physiological presence was a large energy in between my shoulder blades. In the moment of recognition, that energy turned into light and rose like a grail into Divine love and mercy. I knew then that Sadguru knew everything about me and had my situation in full control, and that I needn't worry anymore."

W. H., Crestone, CO

Commentary: The power of Divine compassion is infinite and without judgment. Such cleansings are a direct gift of the link of the Lord of Lords to anyone who practices this mantra.

✖

"I heard a voice coming from inside me, 'You are so close!' Then I saw the Elephant God, Ganesh, the remover of obstacles and Lord of new beginnings. He was blue and said for me to let go of all my attachments. So I bowed and let go of everything. Then an orange-clad yogi put one hand on top of my head and his other hand under my chin and said, 'It is time to speak what you most deeply desire.' And I said, 'Ultimate fulfillment.' Then I saw a great rainbow, a gateway, and I went through it into a lake of Pure Consciousness. Then I was guided to enter, which I did. And finally a fish showed me how to swim in these waters, and I became a fish and swam. And then I experienced some pain in my solar plexus and heart."

T.L., St. George, UT

Commentary: Inward journeys are not uncommon in terms of the vast range of experiences with this mantra, and some inner sojourns are marvelously dramatic and inventive, yet even the most imaginative events are meaningful and revelatory. Here, this marvelous voyage is correlated with an effect in the third and fourth chakras, showing that what is happening in the mind has definite physiological correlates, and that the willingness of this aspirant results in the excellent gift of purification.

※

"The thing I find most remarkable still is the experience I had at the ashram where I was doing many *malas* a day. I went into meditation and then extraordinary waves of bliss started pouring through my body. And then it turned into what I can only call 'God intoxication.' Then I lay down and a ball of light began to, seemingly with intention, move through my body very systematically to areas that needed healing. This lasted over an hour. What was most interesting was the feeling of no limitation to what this mantra can do. What I'm left with is the flavor and sense and grace of the mantra to heal on levels that have zero to do with the overtly conscious mind."   B. H., Crestone, CO

Commentary: Such an experience, by virtue of the beauty and love that were here communicated, heal at deeply subtle levels and in equally nuanced ways. There is no limit to the beauty and love that a human being can experience— because there is no limit to the beauty of the Supreme. The blessings of mala jaapa are very real.

※

"It was my second exposure to this particular meditation and, though my first experience was a very moving and powerful one, it was nothing compared to this. ...Chanting the mantra, over and over again, I had some resistance in letting myself go at first, but it wasn't long before I surrendered my egoic identification and just became the mantra.

My body began to resonate with the mantra, to vibrate the energy within me to the point where I no longer could distinguish where my body stopped and everything else began, which lasted until we finished chanting the mantra. In meditation, with my eyes opened, as I always meditate, I began to see the entire room filled with colored lights: ...red, then orange, then yellow, then green, then grayish blue, then blue, and finally purple. Finally, the room illuminated into the most beautiful and brightest color of Orange Light I have ever seen...breath-taking...infinitely wondrous with a feeling of "Presence"...like an infinite blessing, as if the Divine filled me with Presence. The Stillness felt very full, as if an over-abundance of Something wonderful was pouring into me, like water into a balloon. I felt as if Divinity Itself was pouring Itself into me. During all of this, I kept hearing what seemed to be a Whisper, yet It wasn't inside of me nor outside of me.... It was in everything and everything was in It and It kept calling and repeating the name "Shiva", over and over again, very slowly and very softly but very powerfully, yet peacefully...directed completely and utterly at me. It was like the voice began filling me with even more of this stillness, fullness and bliss. The voice was there...until we came out of the meditation. There are really no words that I can use to describe It. It was the most peaceful and harmonious voice I had ever experienced. Since that experience, I cannot explain how I am. I just Am. Everything became clear and still. Everything just Is."   S. S., St. Louis, MO

Commentary: Whether we come to this mantra as novices or are ready for more advanced studies, this mantra will support us wherever we are. Its support is dynamic, such that we are always being moved into our next 'step'. However, we step as we wish, for the choice to journey onward is always ours.

※

"I spent most of my adult life battling and suffering with depression due to the effects of negative thinking. When a friend...told me about this mantra, after my usual period of resistance and doubt, I slowly, reluctantly and heartlessly began trying it out. I struggled along for months with my ups and downs. Until one day I asked myself, "What have I got to lose?" and decided to just let go a bit. I actually chanted...without my usual doubt and cynicism, but with my heart. I now can say that it works. *Hari Om Tatsat Jai Guru Datta* is a powerful grace. My heart opened and peace came in...beyond the madness of mind. It has given me so much these past five years."   S. E., Lebanon, NH

Commentary: Reluctance and skepticism are no barriers to receiving the blessings of this mantra. Doubt requires some degree of persistence. There is great value in persistence but, when sincerity enters, then the Lord's longing for our beauty and freedom meets our conscious recognition of wanting more from life...and that 'more' announces itself and starts to marvelously unfold.

※

"When the *Hari Om mantra* came into my life, I was in the thick of a midlife crisis. My husband and I had just given up trying to bring a child into our lives after many years of trying to conceive and then also ruling out the option of adoption. So what was my purpose as a woman, if becoming a mother was *not* what was in store? This was an extremely painful and difficult time.

During my to my first *Dhun* with Bapu during his visit to the U.S, I had a vision of myself as a ball, hopelessly wound up in layers upon layers of string. The message was: 'You have created this and only you can undo this.' I cried almost the whole evening, overwhelmed at this reality.

As the next few days passed, now in retreat with Bapu and about a hundred others, I was blessed with my deepest prayer—to simply surrender to the Divine Mother. I just let go during meditation. 'Mother, take me!' I cried. Watching over me at every moment, She took me through what I later learned were called *Kriyas:* endless tears, spontaneous *asanas* and hand *mudras,* deep *pranayamic* breathing, visions, 'wild' moans and expressive circular movements in my body, arms and face—all of which I had no control over. At first, it felt like I was "giving birth"—a very 'juicy' physical experience. My nights were spent in a state of trembles and feverish rest. I dreamed it was my birthday, eating a big piece delicious chocolate cake! There were friends celebrating with me. Golden napkins glittered in the background. So much of the sweetness that I had denied myself up to now, was finally here for me to enjoy!

I felt happy about this new opening and accepted it

all with gratitude, but still, I wondered, 'What was really happening to me?'

When I finally had the courage to ask, Bapu said: 'This is all about giving birth to your *inner spiritual child.*' No wonder I couldn't conceive a *physical* baby! At that moment I understood. My path in this lifetime was about experiencing the hard labor of giving birth to my *True SELF*! The deep transformative emotional healing was already taking place—on so many levels. Purifying tears kept flowing. I faithfully continued doing the mantra and surrendering to meditation for the months and years that followed. The seemingly endless layers are still being peeled away.

Five years later, still being faced with challenges, the sweet blessings are always there, too: understanding, acceptance, forgiveness and love. The *kriyas*, more subtle now and sometimes different, continue to this day. And there is so much that I simply can't put into words except that the fruits of this path have brought me unbelievable joy, happiness and peace which have overflowed into the lives of my family & friends.

This *Shakti* and *Prana* that I experiences through this *mantra* practice have opened me to my own powerful ways of courage, strength, faith and healing. Even as a long time yoga practitioner, I really didn't understand what the fruits of "yoga" were all about until *Hari Om Tat Sat Jai Guru Datta* came along. *Sahaja Yoga* teaches me so much-- especially humility! Yes, I'm constantly being 're-born'."

E. S. U , Hurricane, UT

Commentary: The life of any individual is unfathomable. All that we have given and received and endured has structured in us the necessity for certain developmental experiences, as well as the gates of release that unlock our deeper abilities to be alive. Hari Om Tatsat Jai Guru Datta brings everything we need, yet only our direct experience with this mantra over a period of time will reveal what an astounding process is actually unfolding... layer upon layer.

"Eight months after I began chanting this mantra, I felt a physical sensation of energy coming into my head. It's been there ever since, pouring throughout my body. Ultimately that energy has brought me peace, which is what I have always longed for. I have been chanting this mantra for 21 years now, and it's a great blessing to have found it. No matter what belief we enjoy or what level we are on, *Hari Om Tatsat Jai Guru Datta* is a great benefit. We are so lucky to have such a tool—to help us find God within us and God without. I will be chanting this mantra for the rest of this life. It has brought me such peace and bliss and guidance—more than I could have hoped for. I was in pretty bad shape when I found it. Now my father has just passed away, and I know he is in God's heart, which is so comforting. Support is everywhere with this mantra. I've never had a lack of anything—guidance, friendship, money—not even once. I have found so much through it—more than I thought was possible."

B. K., Sacramento, CA

Commentary: For those who come openly to this mantra, the Lord is with them in every way. The abundance from such blessings, short-term and long-term, never stops. The Divine energy increases until peace is constant, regardless of the outward events of our lives. "Sadguru never lets go of anyone who comes to this mantra with faith and sincerity," Bapu has often promised.

PART VII

HARI OM TATSAT JAI GURU DATTA IN THE WEST

I am Hindu, I am Jew, I am Jain, I am Farsi,
I am Buddhist, I am Christian, I am Muslim,
I am every religion.

— Bapu —

Introduction

Bapu, the greatest of yogi saints, received the greatest of gifts from Sadguru Dattatreya. Yet, despite the magnificence of its blessings and the vastness of its purpose and capabilities, it is a humble and unpretentious present, indeed. *Hari Om Tatsat Jai Guru Datta* is an easy-to-pronounce mantra which stands as a complete spiritual practice and simply is offered as the finest and most useful spiritual tool the Lord could devise.

While presented to a great personage who is a paragon of the Vedic tradition of India, this gift is a tool for everyone and was given to all humanity. Therefore, its practice in the West is as important and potent as in the East.

Certainly, this mantra spoken by the Lord of Lords represents a universal language whose 'translation' is without loss of meaning or power. Importing this gift from one hemisphere of our globe to the other, therefore, poses no problems and comes freely and authentically.

Yet, getting through the 'customs agent', so to speak, can represent a delicate process. In the practicality of human affairs, we often find that identifications with culture and societal traditions play an important part in people's lives, which is to say that, because this *mahamantra* has been for thirty years practiced primarily in the culture of Mother India, certain ways of expression, observance and devotion have naturally developed, ways that may or may not be meaningful in the West. In every situation there is an opportunity. Thus, the extent to which culture and socialization affect this utterly pure and Divinely spoken gift is the extent to which its appearance in the West can, theoretically at least, represent a renewal of effectiveness.

Hari Om Tatsat Jai Guru Datta has been known in
Europe and the United States since 1982, almost exclusively
due to the efforts of Shanti Vijani. Shantibaba, once an
engineer and a post-graduate student at Massachusetts
Institute of Technology in 1965, was born and raised in the
beautiful western state of Gujarat, India. In the East, he
worked as a designer for nuclear power plants for 12 years,
until he could no longer avoid the voice inside himself
calling to seek a deeper meaning in his life. Returning to
his native India, Shanti set out on his spiritual journey. He
visited all sorts of spiritual teachers, asking, "Can you show
me God?" At some point, he came with a group of people
to Girnar Sadhana Ashram and saw Swami Punitachariji
(Bapu). It was here that Shanti heard the *Hari Om Tatsat
Jai Guru Datta mahamantra.* Bapu didn't even look at
Shanti, yet did mention that, if one really wants to grow,
an *anusthan* (52 *malas* of *jaapa* a day for 52 days) would
be advisable. So Shanti went home, a few hours away,
and did the 52-day practice, which changed him forever.
Within a few short months Shanti says he noticed, "The
doors to myself remained open." He was on fire to teach
everyone this practice which had reaped such fruits in his
life, at times driving 300 miles if even a single person was
interested. Shantibaba has a gift of translating this practice
and his experiences to the west. He has served as a guide
for thousands of seekers of all faiths with a special gift for
transmitting the mystical energy of spiritual awakening.
In 2000, he initiated the formation of The Tripura Yoga
Foundation. He currently travels nationally as TYF program
leader and makes his home on Maui, Hawaii.

The Definite 'Pathless Path' of *Sahaj Dhyan Yoga*

You know the road I travel,
Every stone and pothole, even the scurrying of the ants.
I know You know the placement of each of my steps.
Which is how I keep both eyes on You
*   and worry not a whit for where my foot will fall.*

—Vishnu Datta—

Even in the Vedic tradition of Hindu India, the tradition out of which this *mahamantra* arises is one which rather defies description.

Bapu—now both a *dende swami* (the highest order of renunciate) and in the *rishi* tradition (of Vedic seers) as a father and family man—is in the lineage of the *Navanaths* (the Nine Masters) who are considered the greatest of souls and closest to Sadguru Datta. Bapu, Maharishi Shri Punitachariji, is understood to have been Gorakshanath, the second of the Nine *Naths*, who took birth some 1000 years ago. His master, Machendranath, who brought *hatha yoga* to the planet and is the first of the Nine *Naths*, was said to be the greatest of all teachers, for he made his disciple Gorakshanath, greater than he himself was. The Nine *Naths* are considered to have the most intimate possible access to the Lord of Lords.

The tradition of Lord Dattatreya is referred to as the *avadhoot* tradition. There is only one real *avadhoot*: The Guru of Gurus. Yet a human being can attain a *sahaj* (natural) depth of enlightenment that such a soul, as Bapu, becomes incapable of doing anything other than the moment-by-moment will of the Divine. *Avadoots* are so selfless as to allow the Lord to work through them purely. Moreover, they are generally solitary saints, certainly not ones to start a publicly visible movement or enact an international vision. Thus, Bapu is quite innovative, for an *avadhoot*.

As already mentioned, Lord Datta appears generally as a madman or a farmer to those fortunate enough to see Him in our human reality. Here, again, we see a focus on consciousness, on penetrating intimacy, on transmission, on going beyond expectation and cultural conditioning— which is characteristic of the way of Lord Dattatreya and the way life works around this mantra. Again, this mantra is not for the masses, not for those who want to be like others, but for souls who want to be extraordinarily and vastly (yet humbly) themselves. The great Datta *avatars*, like Bapu, usually have had devotees from more than one spiritual tradition—mainly both Hindu and Muslim. At Girnar Sadhana Ashram it is common to see Jains, Seiks, Christians, Buddhists, Muslims and, of course, Hindus of every description.

This mantra—in itself empty of rituals, over-riding philosophies and the dos and don'ts of dogma—carries the *avadhoot* energy in so far as there are no rules, except to use it faithfully.

With no particular handles to hold onto—no pews or stained-glass windows or hymnals or dress codes or churches or catechisms or official priesthood or seminary or organization of communities or hierarchy of elected representatives—the grasp of this practice comes inwardly through the graces of the practice itself. Therefore, it has been called "the path of the Yogi mystics," for all we need and all we have is ourselves and our relationship with the Lord of Lords, and our use of this *mahamantra*. Bapu emphasizes the need for faith—faith in God, faith in the mantra and our practice, and faith in ourselves.

Many spiritual lineages and ways refer to themselves as a 'pathless path,' meaning—when an aspirant, moving beyond the limitations of culture and society and family and even religion, is finding the reality and fullness of life in the present moment—that the notion of 'path' becomes less and less a relevant image for one's journey to fulfillment. Yet, with *Hari Om Tatsat Jai Guru Datta* and this 'pathless path' of *sahaj dhyan yoga*—the Yoga of Spontaneous Meditation— there is a noted difference. While 'pathless', this path is nevertheless definite. It is definite because we know what to do: we simply keep faithful to and confident in this mantra and use it regularly. The Lord has made our way elegant. Not that all challenges will be removed, but that we have a simple practice that brings us all that we require.

Sahaj dhyan yoga—the Yoga of Spontaneous Meditation—leads us both uniquely and universally to fullness, a fullness that is whole yet never before expressed in the way we each will enact it. *Sahaj* means that everything will feel natural and that whatever we need will find us, spontaneously—all we need will come without our making any unnatural effort. The Lord knows what we require and wants to give to us, and thus the name 'Datta': the one who gives everything away. *Dhyan* refers to Spontaneous Meditation, such that we are moving as rapidly as possible in peace and purification toward the infinite. And *Yoga*, which means 'union', continually links our individual journey to the unlimited state of freedom and moves us toward that unity, the state of non-separation which culminates our sojourn of spirit and is the goal of every human life.

Sahaj dhyan yoga leads to the highest and most integrated state of human beingness.

Beyond Cultural Interpretation

Many are the beauties I walk through—
The dress of the water carriers, the palace guards,
The local spice on my tongue at the marriage ceremony.
But even the perfume of lovers I would give up for pure love.
                                                    —Vishnu Datta—

Without a theology or organization to oversee the
spreading of this mantra, *Hari Om Tatsat Jai Guru Datta*—
while fitting easily into the Hindu-Vedic context—does not
in itself require such identification. The Datta invocation,
the Datta Vandana and the Datta Stutti (presented in the
Appendix), for example, though beautifully addressing the
Reality that is Sadguru and this mantra—are not requirements
for full benefit with this gift given through Bapu to the world.

There are a great number of souls in the West of
Indian origin, and for many of these individuals the traditions
of Hindu culture and the Vedic tradition—truly one of the
great spiritual rivers of our planet flowing into the Ocean of
Being—are and will be deeply meaningful. Indeed, we are
each invited to have our own relationship with this mantra
and its practice of Spontaneous Meditation. If we wish to
participate in the ways of relating to this mantra which have
already developed, whether or not we are drawn to the Hindu/
Vedic tradition—then excellent. Or if we naturally find
ourselves developing our own accoutrements that bring us
uniquely closer to ourselves and to our practice through this
mantra—then also excellent.

In the interests of purity, truth and the authenticity of
self-development and Self-Realization, let us be clear that

culture—no matter how engaging or time-honored—has its limiting factors. By not assuming the necessity of the cultural contributions that in India have surrounded this mantra since 1975, the potential for the power and depth of *Hari Om Tatsat Jai Guru Datta* in the West are theoretically improved, simply by the fact of moving beyond image and ornamentation to that purity of relationship without any distraction whatsoever. Again, whosoever feels the need and is drawn to ritual and devotional observance, it is in the best interests of such souls to utilize any such practices that will assist in developing sincerity and intensity. As long as we are each free to use or not to use any given practice or custom, this mantra will continue under the direct supervision and grace of the Guru of Gurus.

In any event, *Hari Om Tatsat Jai Guru Datta* in the West has the potential of a deep and abiding purity and potency in all open hearts.

What Gets Released Beyond Image

I came to you because of the luminescence of your smile,
The way you danced round the fire, mad and free,.
Your humor, your culinary zest, your talent at swordplay.
Having seen your heart, I can only kneel
>   *in the empty chapel of love, and I am ready*
>   *to give up even that.*

—Vishnu Datta—

Any image—no matter how real, beautiful, ornate or costly—can only hint at the Reality that the image symbolizes, whether it be a word or a law or a *murti* (statue) or a painting or a photograph or a temple. The Essence is hidden, is more underground than the roots of a tree, is pure mystery. To the extent that an image reveals the mystery, it is a benefit to those who can move to Essence through image. However, history is replete with examples of image losing its status as mirror and the Essence through the image being lost due to a lack of reverent subtlety in the attitudes of those interested in such an image.

The principle, again, is that what is more subtle is more powerful, creative and intelligent than what is less subtle. Though our five senses gravitate to what has shape, weight, texture and color, what is essential is far more beneficial and transformative than what is gross, no matter how lovely to the eye. Thus, this mantra itself, without cultural overlay, can potentially be enjoyed in its purity, without intermediary of any sort, such that results with this *mahamantra* may well be enhanced here in the West.

How This Mantra Spreads

The abandon of children leads me
Secretly to play in fountains.
There is no manual about such frolic, no organized
      movement of children.
One simply sees what one loves and jumps in.

                    —Vishnu Datta—

    This mantra is the most complete of mantras, the most protected and innocent. In its very nature is the encoding of its propagation. Thus, word of mouth from heart to heart is the principle river of *Hari Om Tatsat Jai Guru Datta.* Retreats, at least a weekend, are the preferred venue, since Bapu at his ashram at the foot of Mount Girnar has said that it takes at least three days to grasp this mantra, that he cannot give all that is required in just one encounter.

    Since this mantra is easy to pronounce, can be easily imparted, has no secrecy codes and yields results automatically, anyone who has experienced this mantra can offer it to someone else. Individuals can offer this mantra in a context of Spontaneous Meditation in their homes. Giving retreats does, however, require deep experience and training, since the experiences which arise will bring the necessity of wisdom, compassion, faith and strong knowledge.

    One note: This mantra is what it is and nothing else. It is unitive and its directness from the Lord, Who upholds all His creations, is universal. Thus, this mantra per se has no allegiance to social conformity or political persuasions. Individuals who come to this mantra well may have important social, political, economic, educational or religious beliefs and visions—and their use of this mantra may well support their good works. Yet this mantra in itself does not acknowledge favorites—neither in individuals nor in actions. *Hari Om Tatsat Jai Guru Datta* is apolitical and in every case neutral, being common to all persons and causes.

   If you do come to enjoy this *mahamantra* and wish to share it, please do so. If you wish to contact the author for any question about the use of *HariI Om Tatsat Jai Guru Datta*, the invitation is definitely extended.

Community

I am the horse returning to the barn a bit faster than I left.
The mystery is too deep to hold alone.
Come and let us speak together
Of the glories in the waving of our manes, of all the ways
our hooves are touching the ground.

—Vishnu Datta—

The demands of our times suggest more and more with each passing year the need for community, for working together, for that harmony which is more than the individual notes that expresses the mystery of relational synchrony.

Many wise persons have predicted that the key to the future of our human family, especially in the difficult times of global transition, lies with small communities.

The assembly of like-hearted souls significantly increases the power and expansiveness generated through *sadhana* so that its effects are magnified. Moreover, souls sharing a spiritual path support one another, such that their shared energies add up in ways that are mutually supportive, thereby quickening the pace of their journeys and deepening their experiences.

Bapu has called those who value this mantra "a family" and encourages us to share and participate in one another's joys and sorrows. He is pointing to the great value in relationship, and the unparalleled opportunity for growth that relationships provide. The tie of this family is of the deepest order, and the potential for connection at other levels of interaction is unlimited.

The intrinsic urge toward community is a motion that

may well be a cornerstone in the growth and service of all *sadhaks* (those who perform *sadhana* with this *mahamantra*), as well as a model for relational society for the world—as a communal extension of the Divine gift of *Hari Om Tatsat Jai Guru Datta.*

It is time that the world has examples of souls living together in the energy, knowledge and service that constitutes true community and represents Heaven on Earth. Our human family needs the inspiration of groups of individuals assembling around the deepest longing of their hearts.

Contacts

Swami Vishnu Datta

Mailing address:	P. O. Box 332
	Crestone, CO 81131
Email:	sancthse@amigo.net
Phone:	(719) 588-4257 [cell]
	or (719) 256-4420 (Sanctuary House)
Website:	www.jaigurudatta.org
	www.sanctuaryhouse.org

Tripura Yoga Foundation

Phone:	(808) 280-1339 [Shantibaba's cell]
Website:	www.tripurayoga.org

Datta Yoga Mission Europe

Mailing address:	4 Malvern Road
	Thornton Heat
	Surry CR7
	England
Email:	DattaMission@BlueYonder.co.uk
Phone:	44-2086831333

Girnar Sadhana Ashram and Bapu:

Mailing address:	Bhavnath Taleti, Dattatreya Road
	Junagadh 362 004
	Gujarat
	India
Email:	dattaad1@sancharnet.in
Phone:	(95285) 2624547
Website:	www.sahajyoga.org

Appendix

Introduction

The *Hari Om Tatsat Jai Guru Datta* mantra, though complete in itself, has for years been traditionally accompanied by an Invocation which describes the source of this Divine revelation, its glory and goal. The *Datta Stutti* and the *Datta Vandana* describe the oneness and centrality of Lord Dattatreya by indicating that all the Divine incarnations and power of the Godhead are forms of Sadguru Datta. Such practices, while not in any way requisite for the benefits of this Supreme gift, have definite beauty.

THE INVOCATION
HARI OM TATSAT JAI GURU DATTA

OM [Sung three times]
     and/or
OM GAM GANAPATAYE NAMAH

I bow to Lord Ganesh [remover of obstacles & giver of prosperity] ['Gam' is a bija mantra, a sound particular to and sacred to Ganesh. 'Ganapataye' is a name of Ganesh.]

AKHANDA MANDALAAKAARAM

VYAAPTAM YENA CHARAACHARAM

TATPADAM DARSHITAM YENAA

TASMAI SRI GURAVE NAMAHA

The unbreakable wholeness [or completeness]
Which covers the entire creation:
To the One who shows me that,
To such a Guru I bow

AGNAAN TIMIRAANDHASYA

GNAANAAN JAN SHALAAKAYAA

CHAKSHURUR MILITAM YENA

TASMAI SRI GURAVE NAMAHA

When ignorance pervades the world,
The Wise One comes
And puts the Light of Wisdom in our eyes:
To such a Guru I bow

GURU BRAHMA, GURU VISHNU

GURU DEVO MAHESHVARAHA

GURU SAAKSHAATH PARABRAHMA

TASMAI SRI GURAVAI NAMAHA

I bow to that magnificent Guru who himself is
Brahma, Vishnu, & Maheshvaraha [Shiva],
[Creator, Preserver, Destroyer]
Who when combined together is the Supreme Absolute:
To this type of Guru I bow

GURUR MADHYE STHITAA MAATAA
MAATRU MADHYE STHITO GURUHU
GURUR MAATAA NAMASTETU
MAATRU GURU NAMAMYAHAM

My Guru is my mother
My mother is my Guru
To both my Guru & my Mother I bow

BRAHMAANANDAM PARAM SUKADAM
KEVALAM GYAANAMURTIM
DVANDVAATITAM GHAGANA SADHRUSHAM
TATVA MATSYADHI LAKSHYAM

Salutations to the Guru, the Brahman, who is bliss,
who is the giver of supreme happiness,
who is the Absolute, who is Knowledge personified,
who is beyond the pairs of opposites, who is infinite like the sky,
who is the goal of the Vedic assertions like "Tat-Twam-Asi,"
   [*Thou Art That*]

EKAM NITHYAM VIMALAMACHALAM
SARVADHI SAAKSHIBHUTAM
BHAAVAA TITAM TRIGUNA RAHITHAM
SADGURUM TAM NAMAAMI

who is One, Eternal, Pure & Changeless,
who is beyond the grasp of the mind,
who is beyond the three qualities of nature. [Gunas]
To Sadguru I bow:

ASATOMAA SATGAMAYA

TAMASOMAA JYOTIRGAMAYA

MRITYOMAA AMRITAMGAMAYA

AAVIRAADHIM YEDHI

> The one who takes us from untruth to Truth,
> The one who takes us from darkness to Light,
> The one who takes us from death to immortality,
> from half-truth to Truth.

TWAMEVA MAATAA CHA PITAA TWAMEVA

TWAMEVA BHANDUS CHA SAKAA TWAMEVA

TWAMEVA VIDHYAA DHRAVINAM TWAMEVA

TWAMEVA SARVAM MAMA DEVA DEVA

> Thou art my Mother, my Father Thou art,
> Thou art my Brother, my Friend Thou art,
> Thou art my Knowledge.
>> [the very thing which I am learning inside]
> My Wealth Thou art,
> Thou art my Everything, my Light of Lights

OM SHANTI SHANTI SHANTI

> [Peace, peace, peace]

THE DATTA VANDANA
(Prayer to Sadguru)

DATTA DIGAMBAR VISVA SWARUPA
ANANDA SAGAR AVADHOOT RUPA
ATMA SWARUPE JE PRAKASHMARA
SRI SAGURUNE VANDAN HAMARA

> Datta is the one who gives us knowledge and wisdom.
> With sky for clothing, the Universe is her/his form
> Datta is the ocean of joy and intoxicated union with Reality.
> The one shining in our heart as Self—to that Sadguru I bow.

NIRGUNA NIRMULNE SADA UPAKARI
BHAKTO PAREJE NIJHITAKARI
SRAGUNA SWARUPE SIKKA APANARA
SRI SAGURUNE VANDAN HAMARA

> Sadguru is without the three *gunas*
>   [creation, preservation, destruction]
> Always compassionate, ready to help otherswhen in need—
> Especially devoted souls. S/he has no form,
>   but appears in form to guide seekers.
> To that Sadguru I bow.

ADRISYARUPE DUDHAMACHE GHEE
SAAGARMA LAHERO CHANDANMA AGNI
BHRAMANDA JEMA VISVA ADHARA
SRI SAGURUNE VANDAN HAMARA

> Secretly, just as ghee is hidden in milk,
> Fire is hidden in sandalwood,
> Ripples are always hidden in the ocean,
> In the same way, Sadguru is hidden everywhere
>   in the entire universe,
> And to that Sadguru I bow.

     From The Mouth Of The Supreme

EE RANAKRISHNA BRAHMANE VISHNU
MAHADEVA SHAKTI SURYA GAJAMAN
VIDHVIDHRUPE WAHE TEJDHARA
SRI SAGURUNE VANDAN HAMARA

> Sadguru is Lord Ram, Lord Krishna,
> Lord Brahma, Lord Vishnu
> Lord Shiva, the primal power of life,
> the Sun, the remover of obstacles.
> All is Sadguru's form—just as electricity can take different
> forms, As light, heat and power. To that Sadguru I bow.

BHAKTONI CHINTA HARNARA JE CHE
DEHABHYAN BHULI FARNARA JE CHE
ANTANKARANANE JE UJALANARA
SRI SAGURUNE VANDAN HAMARA

> Saguru is the one who removes the worries of the devotees.
> S/he roams without body consciousness,
> The one who shines in our inner heart,
> removing the impurities.
> To that Sadguru I bow.

HE MUDH CHITTA HAVE JAGIJANE
PARABRAHMA PRABHUNE SARANE TU JANE
GRAHI HATH JE CHE BHAVA TARNARA
SRI SAGURUNE VANDAN HAMARA

> Oh dense, foolish mind, awake, awake!
> Wake up and surrender in freedom to Sadguru, the one
> Who holds your hand to cross the ocean of worldly
> illusion to the other shore.
> To that Sadguru I bow.

THE DATTA STUTTI

This dhun (chant) salutes Sadguru Dattatrreya as being the Source of all divinity, such that all the Gods and Goddesses and Divine incarnations are the form of the Lord of Lords.

NIRANJANA SWARUPA   JAYA GURU DATTA
    [God in a form]
NIRAKARA RUPA   JAYA GURU DATTA
    [God without a form]
HARI OM TATSAT   JAI GURU DATTA

VISHVA SWARUPA   JAYA GURU DATTA
    [All that is]
PARABRAHM RUPA   JAYA GURU DATTA
    [and all that is beyond]
HARI OM TATSAT   JAI GURU DATTA

BRAHMA SWARUPA   JAYA GURU DATTA
    [Lord Brahma]
NARAYANA RUPA   JAYA GURU DATTA
    [Lord Vishnu]
HARI OM TATSAT   JAI GURU DATTA

MAHADEVA RUPA   JAYA GURU DATTA
    [Lord Shiva]
JAGADAMBE RUPA   JAYA GURU DATTA
    [Mother Divine]
HARI OM TATSAT   JAI GURU DATTA

ISHU SWARUPA	JAYA GURU DATTA
[Jesus]	
ALLAHA RUPA	JAYA GURU DATTA
[Allah]	
HARI OM TATSAT	JAI GURU DATTA

BUDDHA SWARUPA	JAYA GURU DATTA
[Buddha]	
MAHAVIRA RUPA	JAYA GURU DATTA
[Mahavir (Jain Avatar)]	
HARI OM TATSAT	JAI GURU DATTA

TU HI RAMARUPA	JAYA GURU DATTA
[Lord Rama]	
TU HI SHYMRUPA	JAYA GURU DATTA
[Lord Krishna]	
HARI OM TATSAT	JAI GURU DATTA

BHAKTI SWARUPA	JAYA GURU DATTA
[All that is devotion]	
SHAKTI SWARUPA	JAYA GURU DATTA
[All that is power]	
HARI OM TATSAT	JAI GURU DATTA

SIDDHA SWARUPA	JAYA GURU DATTA
[The perfected beings]	
AVADOOTA RUPA	JAYA GURU DATTA
[Those beyond selfhood]	
HARI OM TATSAT	JAI GURU DATTA

HARI OM TATSAT	JAI GURU DATTA
HARI OM TATSAT	JAI GURU DATTA
SADGURU DEVAKI JAI	

About The Author

Teacher, poet, retreat master, and philosopher, Swami Vishnu Datta (William Howell) has studied with adepts since 1971. His teachers, all inter-religious in their own right, have included Maharishi Mahesh Yogi, Sheikh Nur al-Jerrahi (Lex Hixon), Father Thomas Keating and Shri Punitachariji Maharaj (Bapu). In 1994, William became a builder, founding and for nine years constructing Sanctuary House, "an inter-religious retreat center in the round," located in Crestone in Colorado's San Luis Valley, at the foot of sacred mountains. William is Yusuf Anwar al-Jerrahi, a khalifa in the Nur Ashki Jerrahi Order of Sufis since 1988. He received the Hebrew name of Abraham Ben Torah in 1979, and entered the Roman Catholic Church in 1986 with the confirmation name Francis, after Francis of Assisi, who is the patron saint of Sanctuary House. In 1996, he took refuge as Karma Zopa Gyurme with the late Bhokar Rinpoche. In 1997, he met Bapu at Girnar Sadhana Ashram in India at the foot of sacred Mount Girnar. In 1999, when Bapu came to America, William received the name 'Vishnu Datta'. In 2001, Bapu gave Vishnu Datta *diksha* and made him a swami. Since then, under Bapu's authority, he has been offering the *Hari Om Tatsat Jai Guru Datta* mantra around the United States. Because of his wide spiritual interests, and enjoying inter-religious dialogue, he still gladly answers to 'William' and lives to give all that he has been given.

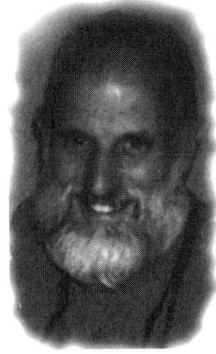